The
Scalpel
and
the Soul

Encounters with Surgery,

the Supernatural,

and the

Healing Power of Hope

ALLAN J. HAMILTON, M.D., FACS

FOREWORD BY ANDREW WEIL, M.D.

JEREMY P. TARCHER/PENGUIN
Published by the Penguin Group
Penguin Group (USA) Inc., 375 Hudson Street, New York, New York 10014,
USA • Penguin Group (Canada), 90 Eglinton Avenue East, Suite 700, Toronto,
Ontario M4P 2Y3, Canada (a division of Pearson Canada Inc.) •
Penguin Books Ltd, 80 Strand, London WC2R 0RL, England •
Penguin Ireland, 25 St Stephen's Green, Dublin 2, Ireland (a division of
Penguin Books Ltd) • Penguin Group (Australia), 250 Camberwell Road,
Camberwell, Victoria 3124, Australia (a division of Pearson Australia Group
Pty Ltd) • Penguin Books India Pvt Ltd, 11 Community Centre, Panchsheel
Park, New Delhi–110 017, India • Penguin Group (NZ), 67 Apollo Drive,
Rosedale, North Shore 0632, New Zealand (a division of
Pearson New Zealand Ltd) • Penguin Books (South Africa) (Pty) Ltd,
24 Sturdee Avenue, Rosebank, Johannesburg 2196, South Africa

Penguin Books Ltd, Registered Offices:
80 Strand, London WC2R 0RL, England

Most Tarcher/Penguin books are available at special quantity
discounts for bulk purchase for sales promotions, premiums,
fund-raising, and educational needs. Special books or book excerpts also can
be created to fit specific needs. For details, write Penguin Group (USA) Inc.
Special Markets, 375 Hudson Street, New York, NY 10014.

ISBN 978-1-58542-615-7

Printed in the United States of America
1   3   5   7   9   10   8   6   4   2

BOOK DESIGN BY AMANDA DEWEY

While the author has made every effort to provide accurate telephone numbers
and Internet addresses at the time of publication, neither the publisher nor the
author assumes any responsibility for errors, or for changes that occur after
publication. Further, the publisher does not have any control over and does not
assume any responsibility for author or third-party websites or their content.

To my wife, Janey—
the sun in my Universe

A good heart . . . is the sun and the moon; or rather, the sun, and not the moon;
for it shines bright and never changes, but keeps his course truly.

SHAKESPEARE, *Henry V*, V.2

Contents

Foreword

Andrew Weil, M.D.

The author of this book is a storyteller and a surgeon. The stories he tells in this book are about experiences he has had through his surgical career, about memorable patients, colleagues, and mentors. Because his specialty is neurosurgery, the patients he has operated on have often come in with devastating conditions, like traumatic brain injuries and malignant brain tumors. They and he faced critical decisions and the imminence of death, with outcomes influenced by the vagaries of chance, luck, and fate.

Allan Hamilton has the whole-person perspective that I emphasize in integrative medicine. Like me, he regards patients as not just physical bodies but also mental/emotional beings and spiritual entities. In order to understand health and illness, doctors must examine and attend to those dimensions of human life as well as the physical, even when the physical body is obviously damaged or sick. The stories you are about to read reveal remarkable interactions between the physical and non-physical aspects of human life as observed by a skilled practitioner and scientist.

Probably many doctors and nurses working in critical care have made similar observations about the influence of emotions on outcomes and the existence of consciousness beyond the brain, but in my experience, few talk about them or let them influence medical thinking and practice. I admire Allan Hamilton for recording and sharing his extraordinary experiences and for drawing useful lessons from them. His conclusions are sometimes surprising and always reassuring, even when drawn from profoundly tragic events.

In addition to performing surgery, Allan has been a surgical patient. Late in life he had to undergo major reconstructive surgery on his lower spine to relieve nerve compression resulting from earlier injuries. The procedure was not entirely successful; continuing pain and weakness in his legs eventually forced him to stop operating. He knows the promises and perils of the scalpel from both ends of it. As a result, he is in a unique position to give practical advice to those of us who will have to decide whether or not to accept surgical treatment, those of us who will have no choice about it, and all of us who contemplate the vulnerability of our bodies and our mortality.

I have known Allan as a friend and colleague at the University of Arizona Health Sciences Center. I consider him credible, grounded, and scientifically minded. Some of the stories he tells are heart-wrenching, some are funny, and some are very much out of the ordinary. I have no reason to question their veracity. They are consistent with my own experience.

I do not have patience with medical experts who dismiss accounts of spontaneous healing and unexpected responses to unconventional treatments as "anecdotes" that are unworthy of scientific attention. "Anecdote" is a trivializing word, used to dismiss observations that challenge the conventional paradigm. Good science begins with uncontrolled observation. If observations do not fit the standard model of reality—especially if they do not fit—scientists should give them attention. They are the raw material from which we form hypotheses to be tested. "Anecdote," by the way, derives from the Greek and means "unpublished." In publishing these "stories from the spiritual side of surgery," Allan Hamilton gives us quite a lot to ponder.

Introduction

The Universe begins to look more like a great thought than a great machine.

SIR JAMES JEANS

This is a series of stories. Every one is inspired by real patients and real events. I have changed little, and where I did it was mostly where it was required to protect someone's privacy. Occasionally, I've protected the identity of a physician who's still alive, primarily for legal reasons. Sometimes I've combined two or more characters.

I started my journey as a doctor trying to understand the differences between the brain and the mind. In the end, I also had to grapple with the conundrum of the soul. In part, this is a series of stories about becoming a physician. It is also about finding myself unprepared to wrestle with spiritual questions and crises I encountered. There was, inevitably, a reckoning. I had to reassess my life, from childhood to the present, from my own values to those of the patients I met. But this journey is also about redemption. It would lead me to affirmations of life beyond life, beyond death, and beyond fear.

In the early twentieth century, Roald Amundsen, the Arctic explorer, had to pass a winter above the Arctic Circle among the Inuit Indians. He spent the sunless season sharing a dwelling with the tribe's shaman, or medicine man. After months of watching the many sleights of hand and minor tricks the shaman used to hold the attention of the tribe with his magic powers, Amundsen could no longer restrain himself. He decided to confront the shaman and ask him: Didn't it bother him that all his "magic powers" were nothing but cheap parlor games? The shaman smiled. He replied, "My magic power is not in my tricks. My real power is that I have gone out on the ice and lived there alone for many months until I could finally hear the voice of the Universe. And the voice of the Universe is that of a mother calling after her beloved children. That is my real magic."

I hope there is some real magic in these stories too. I'd ask you to symbolically take my hand and go on rounds as we visit my patients. See them with me at the bedside, as I saw them—then and now. Let them tell you their stories. Let yourself experience their struggles through me. Be patient: their spiritual lessons speak for themselves.

One

Crystal Ball

When I was eight years old, my mom took my brother, Patrick, and me to Coney Island. My mother never would have agreed to take us there if her best friend, Betty, didn't have to go. But Betty had to go because she had a coupon for a 25 percent discount on every child's ticket if the child was twelve or under. Time was quickly running out. Betty's eldest daughter would turn thirteen in a month. So Mom got sucked into going because Betty would not ride the subway alone all the way out to Coney Island.

Just because we were going to Coney Island didn't mean my mom had to like it. She'd never been there but already knew she should hate it. It had a boardwalk. People ate corn dogs and cotton candy. They bought stuffed pandas. They went on rides too. Rides that were good for nothing and went nowhere. Because Mom was of German descent, she distrusted frivolity. Betty, on the other hand, was a devout Irish Catholic and had a grasp of the transience of simple fun.

Betty thought it would be great to find a Gypsy fortune-teller along the boardwalk—someone to read the fortunes of all the children. Mom could scarcely bring herself to hand over the two bits required by the Gypsy woman Betty found. My brother had his palm read first. It foretold he would be rich and marry a movie star. Mom snorted with disapproval. She had a habit of flaring her nostrils when she set herself against something, and they roared open like the air intakes of a jet. But the last straw—the point where Mom just snapped—was when the Gypsy woman took hold of my hand and announced, "This one, he will become a doctor. Maybe even famous." My mother chortled. "Preposterous," she said. She led me out, taking my hand out of the Gypsy woman's.

I was admittedly a poor prospect for a career in medicine. I was frightened of anything remotely organic, like blood or a scab. I could not stand getting my hands dirty. I had other career plans: For the first ten years of life, I had wanted to be a cowboy. This was followed by a two-year stint where I wanted to become the commodore of the SS *United States*. By the time I set off to college, the ship was rusting badly, and I had decided to become a painter instead.

I spent two and half years at Ithaca College trying to master oil painting. While I loved the abundant opportunities to sketch naked women, I couldn't make a go of it. I reluctantly changed to an English major specializing in American literature. A career as a teacher could pay my way after graduation. It offered prospects for a steady (albeit meager) income. But soon even these plans were derailed: I had accumulated enough credits to graduate early—too early!

Premature graduation from college at that time was a terrifying prospect. The Vietnam War was raging. Every young man with a pulse and at least one good eye was being drafted and sent to serve in Southeast Asia. I was in a panic. My draft lottery number was low too: 107. I had a good chance of being called up. I was sure I'd go to Vietnam. I was as good as dead.

I went to argue at the Registrar's Office. There must be some error, I insisted. A miscalculation of credits. How could I be so quickly finished with college? The middle-aged lady at the Registrar's Office smiled at me like a crocodile when I told her my dilemma with the draft. She was quite sure: I would have a dozen more credits than required by the end of the year. And, yes, a note did already go off to my Draft Board. Her delight was obvious. One of the problems with the Vietnam War was almost everyone became an asshole about it.

I went down to the military services recruiting office and sat through days of testing to find out what would prove the best military occupational specialty—MOS—for me. I was never shown the results. They would just tell me to come back the next day for some more exams. There seemed no end to the tests. One of them I really liked: it was an examination where they would check how fast you could move your hands and eyes together. There was another that I really enjoyed: it presented a completely nonsensical language. You had to figure out how to translate the language. I must have done well enough, because right after that test the recruiting sergeant took me aside and asked if I had ever thought about a career in intelligence. You know, like the CIA or the FBI? Well, frankly, I liked those initials a whole lot more than ROV (Republic of Vietnam). So I said sure. Why not? Become a spy, I thought.

Boy, did things change after that. They called me by my first name. Ushered me into a private office. Fetched me coffee. I had to take more tests, but now I was in a room by myself and really giving it my best efforts. There were worse ways to sit out the war, I figured, than working for the government, encrypting and decoding messages. It seemed safe. No bullets required.

So I worked my way up the ladder of aptitude evaluations, IQ tests, psychological profiles, and security clearances, hoping someone would just let me hang out in college.

Then a stoned friend of mine told me about a junior professor in the biology department who worked with birds of prey. This guy was looking for a lab assistant, my friend claimed.

"Yeah, so? What does this guy have to offer me?"

"Well, man, this prof, he's like training these birds of prey to swoop down and kill pigeons so they can't get sucked into these mother Air Force fighter jets."

"He's killing pigeons?"

"Well, it sure beats killin' babies!"

"Sure. Sure. I know what you mean." I really didn't, but try arguing with someone who's completely stoned.

"Well, wake up!" my friend shouted. "He's training these birds for the Air Force! Every time, he like takes out one of his hawks, and puts a hit on a pigeon, well, that 'whack' saves Uncle Sam millions by making sure those birds don't get sucked into the jet and crash it. Man, these motherfuckin' hawks are worth a fortune. Like, this has got to be, like, vital to the national interest or security or something. So a research job like that would have you working at the 'Sneaky-Pete' spy stuff but you could still be in school, like. See? No draft!"

He did have a germ of a good idea there. I'd heard that some research-ers could be spared from the draft because their grants were funded by the Department of Defense. It was worth a shot.

Bruce Denin was an ethnologist whose main research was on bird behavior. His Ph.D. had been on "mobbing behavior," where small birds, such as sparrows or crows, swarm around and literally mob the much larger and more dangerous predatory birds. By flying around in sufficient numbers, and darting in and out, the smaller birds distract the raptor and any chance it might have had to surprise a victim. It struck me as a strange area in which to want to excel as a researcher. It was still worth investigating if it could keep me from being drafted.

The Ornithology Lab at Cornell University was tucked behind one of the long, loaf-shaped hills that overlook Lake Cayuga. There was something promisingly military-looking about the building. It had an entrance with a gate and a guard. He checked your name on a clip-board and phoned ahead. I was encouraged. It smacked of Department of Defense–sanctioned stuff. The building was squat, painted one of those flat greenish-browns from a government color swatch. The whole place practically screamed out "engaged in work essential to national defense"—the key phrase for certain exemptions to military duty.

Dr. Denin was a tall, thin wiry fellow, one half ex–college basketball player mixed with equal parts nerd. He had horn-rims that made his eyes appear large and prominent, like an owl. He also had the birdlike habit of shifting from one foot to the other. Dr. Denin led me into the

"Raptor Building"—row upon row of gigantic flight cages, wire sides rising more than twenty feet in the air. Each cage contained a significant remnant of a tree limb that served as a perch and on each one sat a lone bird. Hawks. Falcons. Some were huge eagles—from Canada, Africa, Asia, and, of course, America. All the birds had been confiscated from smugglers by agents of the U.S. Fish and Wildlife Service.

We passed into one of the flight cages. Once I was inside, I could see it comprised a space of thousands of cubic feet. Still it felt small, claustrophobic. The acrid odor of bird crap didn't make it more appealing. Dried scraps of old meat lay encrusted on the floor.

Our cage was filled with a giant golden eagle, on a corner perch. I instinctively flattened myself against one side of the door, trying to keep my hand close to the exit handle. Dr. Denin squatted down in the center of the cage, and then the massive bird clucked its way over to him like an overgrown chicken, circling on the ground near his feet. Dr. Denin made small kissing sounds. Suddenly the bird hopped up on his arm. It must have weighed well over twenty pounds. I could see the muscles in Dr. Denin's arm straining as he braced himself to support the bird's weight.

At that moment, I would have done anything Dr. Denin asked. I had simply never experienced the majesty and power embodied in that eagle at such close range. So when he sent the bird off to her perch again and asked me to walk with him to his office, I think I might actually have been hyperventilating with excitement.

He explained that he wanted me to undertake a "modest" pilot project with a small passerine bird called the loggerhead shrike. I had never heard of it. The shrike apparently has tiny claws that cannot shred prey. To eat, it must impale its victims on thorns, nails, barbed wire— anything that can be driven into the body to hold it. It sounded like a ghastly trait. Dr. Denin proposed that I work on a research project that involved feeding small mice to a pair of nesting shrikes and then presenting them with an assortment of different-sized nails at different angles in a wooden board to see which "impalement sites" were chosen with the greatest frequency. Not exactly my idea of high-minded science. On a par with discovering which coat hook is preferred most by kindergartners in the cloakroom. But it was research, and slowly it began to matter to me what the outcome would prove to be. I became curious how the shrikes would choose from a seemingly indistinguishable assortment of nails. Eventually, I came to see minute, subtle differences between the nails as far as the shrikes were concerned. I became quite proficient at guessing which spikes the birds would like best. Soon I was batting better than 75 percent.

Dr. Denin complimented me on my progress with the shrikes. He got excited when statistical analysis revealed that nine out of ten shrikes prefer to impale a mouse on a nail jutting out at an angle of 30 to 45 degrees. It isn't the stuff of Nobel Prizes, but maybe it was one new piece of knowledge, and I felt good about having helped to develop it. It wasn't really an ego thing. More a secret, heartwarming feeling—pride that a little bit of humanity's vast store of information bears your little, hidden scratch marks on it.

I guess I got hooked on those shrikes. I was even more excited when Dr. Denin hired me to work in his lab on the main campus. This research involved looking for an obscure protein called antidiuretic hormone (ADH). Its secretion was enhanced by changes in blood volume, and Dr. Denin believed that removing the kidneys in a rat might cause a huge and predictable increase in circulating ADH. It turned out to be a brilliant hypothesis, and eventually led to the identification of a polypeptide hormone called vasopressin, secreted by the brain, now known to be a major determinant of blood flow to the kidneys.

None of this really mattered to me, except that I got to remove hundreds of pairs of kidneys from rats. And boy, did I ever love taking out those kidneys—an operation called a nephrectomy in medical jargon. I loved sitting at the lab bench hour after hour. I enjoyed the feel of the surgical instruments, the press of steel staples, and the dissection of the tissues themselves. My hands began to move faster. My eyes seemed to flash quicker. It was all over: I knew then and there I had to become a surgeon.

I never did get drafted. In that year of 1971 the draft never went higher than 105. But running from the draft helped me discover my own hands. The intellectual side of medicine has never held any appeal for me whatsoever. For me, it's the hands. Getting wrapped up in a quiet, self-sufficient universe stretching between fingertip and eyeball.

Surgeons have a saying: "A day without surgery is like medicine." If you can't operate with your hands, then you lose the quality that distinguishes you from the rest of medicine. Surgery is visceral. Tactile. Being a physician is something else. What else? I can't really say, because I have never wanted to be a physician. Just a surgeon.

My first job after graduation from college was not glamorous: assistant janitor. I cleaned the large Presbyterian church on the main street of Utica, New York. I mopped, polished, and swept that place from top to bottom. I took another job working part-time for a veterinary surgeon by the name of Chris Krasner. He had made me an offer I could not refuse: if I would be willing to work diligently as his "kennel boy," then I could occasionally assist him in the animal operating room suite if my chores were completed.

Being a kennel boy requires more grit than most people imagine. He handles all the dogs. From the sweet ones right up to the big, vicious ones trained as attack dogs. You clean out mountains of feces. Diarrhea. Urine. Vomitus. Hairballs. A tide of organic detritus. The cages and runs need to be ruthlessly disinfected daily. You work with astringents, bleaches, and chemicals that will peel the bark off a tree. You feed all the animals. You bathe and shampoo all those headed home. And when an animal dies, you cremate it. You fire up the incinerator and burn every dead dog and cat to cinders.

Running that incinerator was the most grisly, dirty work I've ever done. If there is a "bottom" from which you are supposed to work your way up, I guess being kennel boy was it. The bodies were all stiff, with malodorous fluids seeping out of them. You'd retrieve all the collars and tags. When everything from each dog was finally burned up, you opened the bottom panel to dig through the ashes. You'd find a scoop that was just clean ash. No recognizable pieces of bone. Then you would put it into a plastic bag, inside a disposable plastic urn, and set it aside along with the collar, the tags, and any toys that might have accompanied the dog. Dr. Krasner would hand this back to the family when they came by to pick up the remains. And pay their bill. Chris was strict about that: you never handed over the ashes until accounts were paid in full.

In exchange for this gruesome assignment, I got to assist Chris with all his surgeries. Chris was widely acknowledged to be one of the best veterinary surgeons in all of central New York State. He did a lot of orthopedic work for hip dysplasia in the large dog breeds like Labrador retrievers or Great Danes. Once in a while we would do abdominal surgery (besides spaying, which was a daily occurrence). Chris occasionally performed a couple of surgeries that really got him excited, and therefore me too. He loved heart surgery, which he only got to do once in a blue moon. And he also loved cataract surgery. Chris was the king of cataracts. It turns out that some breeds are very susceptible to cataracts, especially cocker spaniels. So we always had one or two cockers recovering back in the kennel area. I was very glad that it was not Dobermans that got cataracts. You had to administer ophthalmic ointment into their eyes twice a day, and most cockers were easy to handle. The Dobermans were just plain vicious.

I loved being in surgery every day. I knew I never would have gotten to see real surgery close up any other way. I also knew I wanted to perform human surgery. Not the veterinary kind. Often, Chris would offer an elegant surgical solution to a dog's or cat's problem. The owner would ask how much. Chris would give them a price, and then they would ask, "Well, how much would it cost if we just put him down?" Surgery can never be as cheap as euthanasia. No, I knew that I wanted human surgery, where it was clear from the start that everyone wanted you to perform at the highest level of your skills. And expense was no object—at least theoretically.

Surgery was a kind of sanctuary for me. It met many of my needs and eccentricities. I'm somewhat obsessive-compulsive. As I said, I never like to get my hands dirty. I used to drive my entire family crazy when we would go to the beach. I would stand up for the entire day with my hands held out to my sides so that the sand would not get on me. Surgery's a great field to go into if you want to get clean and stay that way.

Lots of people could get plenty irritated with obsessive-compulsive behavior. You can imagine why. "No, this has to be put over here." And "This always goes back in there." "No, you line them up from the biggest on the right to the smallest on the left." Of course, it could drive anyone out of his mind except in the operating room. I never met a patient who did not want his or her surgeon to be compulsive. So surgery offered me a refuge.

I learned I loved working with my hands, this manually induced "flow state." Like athletes carried away in the moment of competition, or musicians performing a piece of music, surgery carries with it an undeniable, addictive attraction. A flow state that can last for hours. You are completely wrapped up in the work. Time stands still. You don't feel your stomach growling. Or your bladder aching. Or your back groaning. You're hardly aware that the nursing shift has changed, that a whole new team is with you in the OR. You just look up to see that the clock has leapt forward several hours. That is why the operating *room* is called an operating *theater*. Because it *is* a theater—a place of drama. Surgeons don costumes. They put on masks. Then the play unfolds. You can feel the sparks jumping in the air.

When third-year medical students come to see me as a faculty adviser to talk about where to apply for residency and what specialty each of them might consider, I find that the group of students destined to go into surgery are the easiest to counsel. They're the ones who already know that they have no choice: they have to become surgeons. It's simple: if you can't bear to be anything but a surgeon, then you have to go into surgery. Surgery chooses you, not the other way around.

I always think of that old Gypsy woman at Coney Island. Because I've felt that I was drawn into the field of surgery as if pulled by a magnet. Surgery was waiting for me rather than me for it. I would kiss that Gypsy woman now if I could find her. She gave me a secret dose of hope—a shot of mythical confidence.

Two

Ogooué: River of Doubt

n 1981, against my better judgment, I went to Africa as a surgical fellow. My entire being protested against putting my life in jeopardy. To live in the African jungle, cut off from advanced communications, abandoning so much of the surgical sophistication I cherished, seemed like intellectual suicide. But I went. To a small hospital located in the jungle town of Lambaréné (pronounced "Lom-ba-ray-nay"), on the Ogooué (pronounced "Og-goo-ay") River, right on the equator in Gabon.

It was as isolated and ramshackle a hospital as I feared it might be. As a medical facility it had no other claim to fame except that Albert Schweitzer had practiced there as a missionary physician and ethical philosopher for most of his adult life. I thought it might be a professional mistake to go there. What could the primitive Third World teach me that would enhance my surgical career? I was wrong. There I found, the Universe could show an interest in me.

As with Dr. Denin's lab experience, opportunities chose me rather than vice versa. Going to Africa was traced to a childhood fantasy. As a kid, I was a weakling. I was thin. No good at athletics. I was shy. Shortsighted. And had bouts of asthma. My family encouraged me to pursue indoor activities like chess, music, and drawing. My childhood was spent less experiencing life than cataloging it, collecting it from other people's lives—like souvenir buttons, butterflies, stamps, and marbles. And I also worked hour after hour making model ships.

I was an odd recluse. On Saturdays or Sundays, my stepfather would take my brother and me on long walks in the hopes of getting us exercise and fresh air. He always hung a large transistor radio (no smaller than a good-sized bread box) over his shoulder, and we would listen to the WQXR radio station as they played one classical piece after another. The walks would take us to museums and parks around New York City.

By and large, I was reasonably neutral about these "enrichment excursions," as my stepfather called them. He made them sound like bad-tasting vitamins. My brother Patrick loathed them. He had to be dragged kicking and screaming every weekend. I believe Patrick would have happily contracted the plague if it would have spared him from a single weekend outing. By contrast, my timid neutrality struck my stepfather as a ringing endorsement.

The truth is, one of these outings always did leave me breathless with excitement: Sagamore Hill in Oyster Bay, New York. We took a train out there, and I loved that part. But Sagamore Hill itself held me in rapture. It was the rambling home of Teddy Roosevelt, our twenty-sixth and youngest president. I turned into quite a pest and would constantly request returning to Sagamore Hill. My stepfather must have taken me there over a hundred times (bless his heart). As we toured the mansion, he would point out all the ways that TR started off in his life: the way I did mine. He'd enumerate them, first on one hand and then the other. What passed as a litany of my weaknesses now served as links asserting my connection to this heroic and charismatic leader: We were both puny, nearsighted, and asthmatic. Both TR and I collected natural specimens. Both of us were avid readers. Both of us loved ships. And, my stepfather would point out, "Just look at what TR did in his life!" My stepfather gave me something of inestimable value: a hero.

So, almost twenty years after those visits to Sagamore Hill, the opportunity to go on an adventure into the heart of equatorial Africa presented itself. It was that potent, direct inspiration of TR that spurred me to fill out the application. TR would have gone to Africa! He wouldn't have let the parasitic diseases, malaria, and hepatitis stop him. In fact, TR had made a very dangerous and treacherous journey to explore the Amazon basin toward the end of his life, when he was already more than fifty years old. I could speak French fluently, and it gave me a huge advantage in the competition for the fellowship, as that was the official language of Gabon. Again, I was still unaware that an assemblage of coincidences could launch me into new realms of self-awareness.

Before I knew it, I was packed. I had purchased a pith helmet and a khaki jacket. I have to admit that I went down to the Abercrombie & Fitch store on Madison Avenue to shop because that was where TR had shopped for his safari supplies. It was where TR had purchased a custom-made uniform, complete with a colonel's insignia of rank, to embark on the famous military campaign that would take him to that defining moment on the charge up the hill at San Juan in the Spanish-American War. So I went to the town of Lambaréné in Gabon, Africa, because TR would have done it.

The medical responsibilities we were expected to carry out in Gabon ran the gamut from performing complex surgery under rudimentary conditions, to treating bizarre, virtually unheard-of parasitic diseases endemic to the jungle. Our clinical duties included ministering to one hundred souls housed in a forlorn, dilapidated leper colony. A downright bizarre arrangement, as Hansen's disease (leprosy) was entirely controllable by this time with medication. There was no need for isolation or quarantine. But for many of those who had been born and lived inside the leper colony, it was inconceivable to leave, even when the doors to the outside world were flung open in a therapeutic sense. Home—even when it's a leper colony—can be hard to leave.

One of my first assignments was to travel to several distant villages by dugout canoe and get children immunized with the requisite vaccinations during the wet season. For three straight months, during the summer, it rains endlessly. The rivers along the equator become engorged with billions of gallons of water. These torrents provide effective routes to reach the small villages that are isolated for the other nine months of the year. Reaching the children in these villages during that one narrow window of opportunity is vital. Many of them would otherwise die in great numbers from polio, or measles, or chicken pox—diseases we hardly acknowledge anymore as more than a minor nuisance in modern, First World countries of the globe.

The remaining nine months of the year were, naturally enough, called the "dry season." To call these months "dry" is an understatement. More like "crispy." The wild, rushing water that erupted so violently during the wet season suddenly dives deep into the ground. Overnight, roaring currents of liquid mud turn into ponds. A day later, the ponds become puddles. Another day and the mud shatters into dust.

Then not a wisp of moisture is left in the air. Every speck of dust hops a ride on the breeze. For the next eight months, the air becomes blood red, laden with dust particles. Tons of dirt stay suspended on the winds like fine talcum and there it remains defiantly airborne till the rains return a year later, when the red dust is jerked back to earth for another joyride down the river.

At first, this vaccination assignment seemed an easy one. There was, however, the matter of transportation. The vehicle of choice was a small dugout canoe—little more than a large tree that had been crudely scooped out with ax and adze. To one squared-off, wider end was attached a dilapidated outboard engine. I have a bigger motor in my kitchen blender!

Into this boat, I had to load myself, several boxes of vaccine, a dozen syringes, and as many needles. We needed only twelve because we were expected to resharpen the needles on a grinding stone after each vaccination. We then dropped them into boiling water for an hour to sterilize them. So we carried sufficient pots and pans to cook in and to use as autoclaves for sterilization. The grinding wheel itself was a bulky, pedal-operated affair, and the stone that turned on it weighed close to a hundred pounds. I was afraid the stone alone would sink our doubtful dugout. It was a frightful cargo for such a precarious watercraft.

The boat came equipped with a guide: a lean, muscular native from the local Fang tribe named Jean-Michel. He puffed incessantly on Marlboros ("cigarettes Americaines"). To ensure we could go as far as we needed to, we carried two extra five-gallon jerry cans of gasoline. That would give us an extra range of one hundred and fifty miles. Jean-Michel's smoking so near the gasoline made me nervous.

I noticed there was a 30-06 Springfield rifle propped up in the bow of the boat. Jean-Michel informed me the weapon was intended for hippos. I asked if we should expect to run into them on the trip. "Ooooh, *non*, Docteur Alain"—they all liked to use the doctor title but only with your first name. I wasn't even sure anyone in Africa even had a last name. "But sometimes the hippos get quite angry when we pass, and they turn the boat over." The waters of the Ogooué River were unforgiving. There were gravestones in the hospital cemetery, all belonging to white doctors who had drowned on the river.

Sir William Osler, a great teacher and literary giant of medicine, once commented that the personalities of the world were divided into two groups: "roosters" and "owls." "Roosters" are the kind of people who wake up with the sun, jump out of bed, and get their best work done by noon. They hit the sack by eight or eight-thirty, pull the blankets up, and sleep like logs, recharging their batteries for the next day. "Owls," on the other hand, love to burn the midnight oil. "Owls" wait till the world goes to sleep before they sit down and get their best work done. An "owl" sleeps past noon, oblivious to the hubbub of the world's commerce until at least half the day is over.

Jean-Michel's original plan had called for us to leave on a Monday. It would take the better part of a week to make our "aquatic" rounds to the outlying villages. I hoped to get an early start, but Jean-Michel was clearly an owl when it came to rolling out of bed. I was the rooster. For me, the best time of day comes at dawn's first light—one reason I find surgery so appealing. There's nothing like the excitement in the morning as the OR begins to rev up for the day's load of cases. It's an adrenaline rush. In keeping with my rooster nature, I had planned to get our vaccination expedition under way no later than 7 A.M.

The night before, I had gone over the contents of our modest watercraft, taking care to lash everything down so we wouldn't lose equipment and supplies if we capsized. That outcome seemed inevitable, as I beheld our pathetic rivercraft. At the crack of dawn, I jogged down to the river. I was stunned to find "le dugout" was gone.

A faded impression in the sand remained where the boat had once been. I sat down on a log and lit up a cigarette (yes, I smoked too) and waited. When Jean-Michel showed up, I asked him if he knew where the boat had gone. Nope. We would have to find our boat if we were ever going to get vaccinating. Jean-Michel began to scan the visible extent of near and far banks. Probably the boat had washed away during the night. We started walking farther downstream. After more than six hours of wet, grimy meandering, we spotted the dugout, hung up by an overhanging root from an enormous jungle tree that reached into the river. Our fully loaded boat was caught there. It had safely piloted nearly four miles of raging river without a human hand. That suggested a greater seaworthiness than I had ascribed to it.

The outboard engine was gone. By thievery or by accident, it did not matter. Jean-Michel and I proceeded to haul the boat four hundred yards to a small dirt road, where we planned to leave it. But Jean-Michel reckoned it would be wiser to hide it. Back into the jungle we went, covering the boat up with leaves and branches. It was no longer just a boat, it was becoming a curse.

We walked back to the hospital compound in the stifling heat. Just to make things even more miserable, it started to rain. We negotiated with the hospital motor pool to commandeer an old deuce-and-a-half truck, and we drove through the mud back to the jungle. With the downpour, nothing looked the same. It took us hours to find our dugout, so stealthily was it hidden from view. I had so compulsively lashed things into place that it took us more than an hour to undo the knots and load the boat onto the truck.

We rolled back into the compound like two exhausted mariners who'd just landed a giant fish and hoisted it on top of our truck. The rain was coming down in sheets. We had missed dinner too. Then Jean-Michel reminded me we had no outboard motor. We ransacked the motor pool in search of a backup motor. We got lucky: Jean-Michel found one he thought he could fix by morning. I just handed him the keys to the truck, went down to my hut, and drank enough Scotch to fall asleep.

I was certainly no "rooster" the next morning! I was whipped. Dehydrated. Foul-smelling. I tried to wash the sleep from my eyes. Made a halfhearted attempt at brushing my teeth. After swallowing the morning's dose of quinine down with a shot of Scotch, I meandered to the dining hall. I was not about to take on the formidable problems of our dugout on an empty stomach. I must have looked a sight. There was an audible gasp when I came into the dining room.

"We fell in the river," I offered sheepishly. I wolfed down some fruit "compote" (the last thing we needed was a bunch of stewed prunes and apricots to keep our bowels running) and then ate a bunch of "crepes"—some fruit-filled pancakes sprinkled with sugar—and drank some strong local coffee. Then I headed down to see if we could get this immunization expedition on its way.

There, at the river's edge, was our mud-encrusted deuce-and-a-half. On its flatbed lay the dugout, with all the supplies stacked next to it, and what appeared to be a functional outboard. You could tell it had been worked on and freshly greased. Jean-Michel was nowhere to be seen, but I figured from the evidence on the truck bed, he must have worked straight through the night.

I commandeered an assortment of nursing staff, aides, and patients' robust family members to lift our river craft off the truck and retruss it with ropes and halyards. As a precaution, I moved it back from the edge of the bank and lashed the nose to the truck's rear axle. I figured that would be a reasonable anchor.

The hassle of the day before had made me fatigued, and I sat in the shade of a tree and snoozed on and off all morning, intermittently puffing away on Marlboros until Jean-Michel gently roused me. In the blink of an eye, we had undone the rope to the rear axle of the truck, had stuck three paddles (one spare) into the dugout, and were dragging it by the nose down into the muddy current of the river. A small knot of strangers assembled to watch us depart. Jean-Michel settled into the stern, next to the outboard, and I nestled myself amid the provisions in the bow. We shoved off and waved good-bye.

No sooner had we begun paddling away from our little landing area than we shot out into the swirling current. We were off. The whole hospital compound suddenly seemed to jerk back, appearing to fly away behind us. It was clear the Ogooué was in charge. Jean-Michel quickly coaxed the outboard to life, with a couple of pulls of the starter rope. It sputtered, barely whispering above the rush of the water. I wondered why, with all the river's natural acceleration, we needed the outboard, but I quickly saw that paddling was virtually useless. The only way to guide the dugout was with the engine. Jean-Michel did this quite skillfully. The landscape ripped past us in a blur. I could not help but marvel at how incredibly efficient river travel was in comparison to the half-built, half-ruined, washboard roads, the only alternative in the dry season. It made sense that the river had linked the whole network of fishing villages in Gabon for centuries and that the road system remained an afterthought, scarcely worth developing.

I looked back at Jean-Michel. I was feeling anxious, uneasy. He, on the other hand, seemed content, his eyes darting studiously all over the river's undulating surface. He had the rim of a battered Michelin baseball cap low over his eyes, to help with the glare. He wore no shirt, nondescript tan shorts, and flip-flops. One arm was draped casually over the rudder handle of the outboard. Although I couldn't hear the little motor, I could see the rhythmic puffs of bluish exhaust behind us. As I looked at

Jean-Michel, he waved to me, wearing a big smile. He seemed happy to be on the river. I, on the other hand, was already wondering how would we ever make it back to the hospital. I had assumed we would simply reverse our direction and go back upriver. Now it was clear a ride on the river went downstream. Nothing could possibly power us homeward against this current. I suppressed my urge to nag Jean-Michel.

For hours the dugout sped along, taking whatever bends or sweeps the river brought. We didn't stop to eat or urinate. It never occurred to us with such a strong current. It was difficult to talk to each other over the roar of the river and the whining of the outboard motor. We would cup our hands and shout, but, naturally, in our tipsy craft we dared not move closer toward each other to be heard more easily.

"Do you know the way?" I asked.

"What?"

"Where are we going?"

"What?"

"Are we lost, Jean-Michel?"

That one he heard. He shook his head no, and smiled, pointing with the side of his hand along the sweep of the river. We were just going to go wherever this water took us. After half a day, the river finally widened out and took on a quieter, more navigable appearance. Now I could converse with Jean-Michel, and it helped calm me. I was concerned that night would be falling soon. The vegetation along the walls of the river appeared impenetrable. Not only would it put us in dark shadows, there was no breach in the barricade of roots and limbs where we could pull off the water.

"Any idea where we stop tonight, Jean-Michel?"

"There's a flat place about eight kilometers ahead, Docteur Alain. It's a good place. Hippos there. But still a good place," he said.

"How close will we be to the first village?"

"Tan-Beang?" It was pronounced "Ton-Bay-un." He continued. "I don't know. It's down a branch of the Ogooué. I'm not sure. Maybe to the right, maybe to the left."

"You mean you don't know? We're going to come to a fork in the river" (I held my fingers up in an exaggerated peace sign) "and you don't know if we should go right or left?"

He shrugged.

"Jean-Michel, isn't there a map? How are we going to tell which way to go? We'll miss the village, for Christ's sake!"

Jean-Michel frowned at me.

I became overwhelmed with anxiety. No map to guide us. No radio to call for instructions. The fork in the river would soon be upon us. We would be left with flipping a coin or playing "eenie-meenie-minie-mo" for navigation. It occurred to me that this was precisely how individuals got lost in the African wilderness, never to be heard of again. I secretly cursed myself for ever putting faith in my hapless guide.

Soon enough, we came to a relatively straight, open stretch of river, and I could see the fork looming ahead. Both ways looked equally promising.

"Jean-Michel, which way? Left? Or right? Tell me!" I screamed.

He simply shrugged his shoulders again. He really had no idea.

"Let's pull in at the fork. Pull in the boat!" I figured better to pull in to shore than commit to one branch. Jean-Michel didn't seem to care one way or the other. I got the feeling he was just placating my jitters.

Vegetation came right to the river's edge, but there was a small bank of dirt that had been scoured by the current. I pointed to it, and Jean-Michel brought us up alongside. I catapulted myself out and clawed my way up the muddy bank, till I managed to grab the exposed root of a large tree with one hand. With the other, I yanked on the rope tied to the bow.

In that moment, all my frustration with my partner evaporated. I realized how much I needed him. If I got stranded on this bank alone, I was finished. Or he would have to somehow come back up the river for me. I renewed my grip on both the tree and the bowline. Jean-Michel and I were inextricably linked, joined together by the boat, the river, and our journey. One could not succeed or survive without the other.

Suddenly, not knowing where we were seemed insignificant. What mattered was that we were together. I felt a sudden sense of happiness and peace.

Jean-Michel cut the motor expertly as it nosed the boat one final thrust toward our little beachhead. He lunged forward, grabbed the line I was holding, and fell onto me as we tugged the boat to shore. There we were in the mud, both grinning, slimed from head to toe. But we'd landed. We quickly shimmied up the steep shore, hauling the dugout up behind us. Finally, in the midst of a tangle of vines, roots, and moist earth, we rested, lying down, gratefully sucking wind. I slapped Jean-Michel gently on the shoulder. A huge smile broke out on his face, and I knew it came from the heart, as mine did. I felt ashamed about my earlier doubts about Jean-Michel.

As if popped out from the trunk of a nearby tree, a black man, no bigger than a boy, stepped in front of us. There wasn't an ounce of fat on his leathery-looking body. His muscles stood out like cables of ebony steel, crisscrossed with veins. Despite small stature, his physique suggested incredible strength, making me think of a black panther. Our intruder wore only a pair of shorts, and a necklace decorated with a few coins. But a shaggy mass of grayish-white, dense curls gave him a regal appearance. From his shoulder hung a leather sack, inside of which something wriggled. Dinner, perhaps.

It never occurred to me to be scared. He appeared to have no weapons. His thick, calloused feet indicated he'd roamed his whole life without shoes. His hands were, likewise, thick and worn from use. But there was no knife, bow, or gun. He did not even have a staff. He stood looking down at us with an air of kindness, of almost paternalistic love. But he still looked as though he could handle anything.

We both jumped up, wiped our muddy hands, and stuck the right ones out. He stared at it, reached forward awkwardly, and shook it. Jean-Michel made the introductions, first in Fang, and then in French. The old man—if he really was old—answered him in Fang, and then turned back to me, repeating his greeting in French. He glanced down at our little dugout, now beached in the heart of the jungle, with all of its lashed contents. He smiled. There was a suggestion in that smile that we might be the luckiest fools ever to set out on the Ogooué River.

Jean-Michel explained that we were from the Schweitzer Hospital. Did he know the hospital? I wondered. Had he ever been there? Had he perhaps met Schweitzer himself?

"We are looking for the village of Tan-Beang," I explained. "Jean-Michel and I are bringing medicine to the people of Tan-Beang." Our visitor crossed his legs and sat down gracefully right where he stood. He nodded, smiling from ear to ear. Then he took our hands and shook them, this time heartily.

"Yes, I know," he said in broken French. "I thought you would be here yesterday." He shook his head wistfully, as if surprised at his own mistake.

"Yesterday?" I asked.

"I had a dream that two men would be coming to Tan-Beang. That is my village. But in the dream, the two men are lost. They do not know which way to go. So I am asked to stand here and help. I am asked to stand here in the branching place of the river and lead them to my village." He said this simply, factually.

"Who asked you to stand here?" I asked.

"My dream was a message," he said. "But in the dream, you arrived yesterday. I had gotten the message messed up, so I waited. Maybe the dream was right, but I got the days mixed up. Who knows? But you are here!" He beamed from ear to ear.

I was dumbfounded. I remembered all our problems with the dugout. There were no phones, no telegrams, no radios, and no drums. Nothing. There was no way we could have informed him or anyone else that we would be a day late. This man had had a dream that we were coming and that we were lost (which was true enough). He had come to the fork in the river and waited for over twenty-four hours, based on the subconscious instructions from his dream. Why? Then realization dawned: it was not really the waters of the river that carried us. It was the hand of invisible forces. Suddenly, the notion of being afraid, and especially the idea of being lost, seemed absurd.

Our savior's name was David, given to him by French Catholic missionaries who roamed Gabon when it was a colony. His real name, understandable in light of his dream, was Outeen. In Fang, it means "who sees things." The rest of our boat trip with him to Tan-Beang was delightful. Gods could not have been greeted with more reverence and hospitality as we pulled up to the village landing.

When I reflect, finding the village represents the exact opposite of a coincidence—if a coincidence is regarded simply as a random pairing of events. To the impoverished and disenchanted mind, such events would seem coincidental. But I began to perceive that they could also be viewed as intentional. What if Outeen's appearance was meant to occur? What if he had been "willed" to be there? Then it could be seen as a gift. The lesson for me was not so much that we were found and guided to the village. The larger conclusion was that my purpose might be interwoven with a complete stranger's dream, and might even depend on the dreamer, and not on me.

Henry David Thoreau wrote that it was never too late to give up one's prejudices. I accepted the gift. Outeen's conviction that he must wait to lead us to the village had been true. Now events were unfolding as they were supposed to. It was simply undeniable to me that I was "in debt" to his dream. I felt gratitude and relief that something, some force, had sent him to help us.

Jean-Michel and I proceeded from Outeen's village to the next, and the next after that. Eight days later, we had visited over twenty small villages and vaccinated nearly five hundred souls. We finally coasted to a large embankment near the capital city of Libreville. When Jean-Michel pulled our bow out of the water, he began unloading the boat. I was puzzled. "Hey, what are you doing?"

"Unpacking," he answered.

"Why now? Why here?"

He looked at me like I was a complete dunce. "Because we're finished. We're done."

"What?"

Yep. It was the end. Jean-Michel took out the last of our gear and swung the Springfield over his shoulder. We had never seen a single hippo. On the other shoulder, he hoisted our faithful little outboard. With a cigarette dangling from his mouth, he motioned with his chin for me to grab my share of the gear.

I bent down to pick up my duffel bag and a box of equipment. Before I realized what was happening, Jean-Michel gave a hefty kick to the bow of the boat, and off it went into the current, shooting rapidly out of sight.

"Maybe a fisherman will find it," he mused.

"Well, now what? How do we get back to the hospital?"

"Not with a boat," he said. "We hitchhike home."

It dawned on me that the dugouts were a kind of one-way, disposable rivercraft. Next year another one could be built.

"Don't worry," he added. "There's always a ride on the road." Half a mile later, we came to the main road back to Lambaréné and the Schweitzer Hospital and we got a ride.

Some events only gain their true stature when we look back. It's an old woodsman's adage: "If you don't want to get lost, stop and look back over your shoulder to where you've been coming from." Africa had many vantage points like that. At first glance, Africa was impressive as a perspective on Third World medicine and its public health aspects. But as I look back, it was the personal episodes and insights that shook me up and changed me.

It becomes easier to be affected by superstition and the suggestion of supernatural influences when one is immersed in a culture where those beliefs are pervasive. You don't need to be ignorant or illiterate for superstitious beliefs to take hold. The Western assertions about the powers of modern science are just a variation on the theme of deeply held assumptions. It is easy to say you don't believe in ghosts when you haven't seen one. A spell can only be cast effectively on the susceptible. But in Africa, I lost a great deal of my faith in science. I began to have a deeper appreciation for the power of magic, taboos, and curses. How could I explain that a dream sent Outeen to find us at the fork in the river? That our destiny could be so inextricably linked to the reverie of an unknown, unseen stranger? Native folklore could make more sense sometimes than all my Western science.

For example, there's a tale that all the Fang guides tell about a gigantic brown snake that lives at the bottom of the Ogooué River. It's believed to be a powerful serpent that wants to kill white people. When the native guides asked me if I wanted to feel the snake, they instructed me to put my paddle in the water. I would dip the blade of my paddle and feel the current pull at the oar.

"There!" they would say. "That's the snake! He's trying to pull you in so he can eat you." My impression was it was just the current of the river. When I asked if anyone had seen the snake, they all nodded that yes, they had. The serpent, they asserted, could be difficult to see because he was the same chocolate brown as the mud-laden river. Besides, the Fang had better eyes to see the serpent with than the weak eyes given to whites.

Because the snake thirsted to kill whites, the guides insisted that it was crucial to my survival that I never venture out on the river without a native river guide to protect me. Sure, it occurred to me that this kind of superstitious talk helped guarantee that frightened whites always hired the natives to handle the rivercraft. But superstition and folklore take root in fact before they can come into existence. After all, as one of the river guides pointed out, had I not seen all the gravestones of the whites that have died on the river? As I said, there were more than a dozen gravestones in the white cemetery. Almost every one of them had perished on the Ogooué River. So the snake knew when the whites ventured out on the river. A white man could not be too careful in the matter of selecting an experienced Fang river guide, they insisted. All the guides agreed on this.

When I left Gabon and headed back to Boston, I had the opportunity to meet Bob Asher. He had been selected to go to Gabon as the next year's Schweitzer Fellow. Bob had been a year behind me in medical school. He was an avid wildlife photographer and outdoorsman. He had asked me to come over to his apartment in Cambridge and share my photos with him and "brief" him about what he might expect in Lambaréné at the Schweitzer Hospital.

I spent a whole afternoon with him. I shared with him all of my pictures, and some of the stories. I also told him about the great snake in the Ogooué River. I admonished him to never venture out on the river without a native guide. Superstition or not, the Fang guides were experienced rivermen, and their assistance and camaraderie had proven invaluable to me.

Bob, it turned out, didn't take my advice. He was killed going out on the river in a powerboat with a white man from a downstream village to carry out that year's vaccination program. The boat capsized. Both men were drowned. Bob's body washed up thirty miles downstream, two days after the accident. His remains were added to the little cemetery at the Schweitzer Hospital. It may have all been just terrible coincidence, but a little superstition might have helped to save Bob's life.

It's easy to scoff at beliefs in the supernatural when we don't understand their foundations. Magic becomes apparent when the world cannot be negotiated without its application. Then we do need to let ourselves believe. We do. Africa taught me that the supernatural lies just beneath the surface. It only took a small, definite shift in one's vantage point to see it.

As a practicing neurosurgeon, I found it maddening that no matter how assiduously I would hone my personal technical skills, or build my fund of knowledge, I could not overcome the influence the supernatural played every day in my operating room. For example, I learned to never hesitate to cancel a surgery if the patient felt unlucky on that day, or had a premonition of impending death.

Once, I was driving into the hospital to perform surgery when I had to slam on the brakes suddenly because three buzzards were standing in the middle of the road, shredding the carcass of a dead jackrabbit. When I got to the hospital, as my patient was being wheeled into my operating room, I heard his wife lean over him, kiss him on the forehead, and refer to him as "my little bunny." I canceled the case. The warning of the buzzards was not a coincidence. Four hours later, the man suffered a massive heart attack. It probably would have been a fatal one, had it occurred in the middle of my surgery—if I hadn't heeded the warning from those buzzards! Having a myocardial infarction can become a terrible problem under anesthesia.

So which came first? The chicken or the egg? Someone might argue I inadvertently contributed to the heart attack by stressing the patient when I abruptly canceled the case. Or did I save myself and the patient from a disaster? You try to figure it out. I can't.

I had another patient confide in me that he had a dream the night before surgery in which he fell into a lake and drowned. The patient was agitated and I decided to postpone the case. He had terrible chest pain a day later and suffered severe heart failure. For a while, in the coronary care unit, it was touch and go. I remember his cardiologist telling me that he was afraid the gentleman was going to "drown in his own fluids." Just like in the patient's dream.

I can be superstitious about many things going on in the operating room. I pride myself on a low infection rate for my own cases. I am fastidious about all the usual things: scrubbing, changing gloves, antibiotics, and so forth. But I am also superstitious about such details like the number of stainless steel clamps that we place on the scalp to stop bleeding. For me, the final number of clamps always has to be divisible by three, with no remainder. Seems silly, I know. But I always tell my residents about my superstitions, so they count the clips carefully. Once, a resident felt that he did not wish to comply with my request. Unbeknownst to me, the resident had removed a single clamp; that left a remainder of two. A seemingly harmless experiment to overturn a silly superstition.

Bad luck. Bad juju, as I say. The incision became infected two days after the surgery. Later, the resident came up and confessed to me what he had done. I shrugged my shoulders and shook my head in disbelief. I told him, "That was taking a stupid chance—a needless risk, as far as I'm concerned. And one that you had no right to take. It's my patient. And it's my superstitions. And not yours to question!" I don't know why that infection happened, but it's the first and only time I had an infection in a scalp flap.

In the final analysis, superstitions, omens, and intuitions are the reflections of a conscious effort on the part of an individual to detect the subtle signals sent to us from the natural world. If we are convinced that the life and matter around us are mute, then we are confined to the silence of the scientifically concrete. If we are open to subtlety, then the world resonates with significance. A rock tumbles in front of our path because a ground tremor knocked it loose. A hawk alights on the limb next to us because it was looking for prey. Or perhaps the rock was sent to us as a warning and the hawk as a blessing. The black cat. The shattered mirror. The dream. The shadow out of the corner of your eye. Each of us needs to decide: Does or does it not have meaning? We choose. But remember: there's a big difference between a decision and a choice.

Some folk never listen to the little hairs when they stand up on the back of the neck. I listen hard to those hairs. Because they're my intuition speaking to me. There have been countless times when they have helped me save a patient's life. And on more than one occasion, my own.

There's a distinction between a decision and choice. Someone asks you to decide if you want chocolate or vanilla ice cream. You ask for chocolate. Why? Well, you answer, "I like chocolate better than vanilla." But see the difference when you simply state, "I choose chocolate." Why? Simply because I *choose* it. That's how I am about superstition. I *choose* to believe it.

Three

The Dying of the Light

Every parting gives a foretaste of death; every coming together again
a foretaste of the resurrection.

ARTHUR SCHOPENHAUER,

Studies in Pessimism

n my third year of medical school I came upon a terrible secret: I could predict when someone was going to die. There would be a visual warning about when a patient was ready to expire. Usually these premonitions were quite accurate.

It was not a cognitive process. It is also not a pleasant gift, because it's associated with a dark sense of foreboding. When I know an individual is going to die, I am overtaken by a sickening sense of dread in the pit of my stomach, a terrible feeling of inescapable doom. A dark sixth sense.

The secret is simple: a dull, waxy, yellowish light accumulates around those who are about to die. I first appreciated this premonition when my beloved old Labrador retriever, Odin, was dying. I was still working for Chris Krasner and he had been kind enough to do extensive tests and found that Odin was suffering from an incurable abdominal cancer. In a matter of a few weeks he was in enough pain that I was forced to put him to sleep. I noticed that as I held Odin in my arms, and Chris administered the euthanizing solution into his veins, that there was a perceptible change in the light coming from Odin's eyes and face.

At first glance, I suppose, this presentiment about death might have been a silly notion. I think it is telling, however, that I first noticed this phenomenon in animals dying rather than humans. I had never had an earlier awareness of it before this first impression surrounding Odin's death. But I had always been quite keen about animals and felt (and still feel) profound emotional and psychic attachments to animals. Perhaps then I was tuned in more to this psychic linkage surrounding animals dying rather than people.

After my own visual experience associated with Odin's death, I had literally hundreds of occasions to "feel around" for the premonition, and to essentially fine-tune it during subsequent euthanizations at Chris's veterinary practice. Unfortunately, there's hardly a day that goes by in a busy animal practice that veterinarians are not called upon to put as many as a half-dozen creatures to sleep. So I could make use of these repetitive occasions to watch as the animals slipped away, and passed over to the next life beyond. I learned to better focus on my own visceral sensations. I began to notice that there seemed to be some energy or light that spread out from the animals themselves, and then completely enveloped them right before the moment of death arrived.

This energy always emerged, collected, and then departed an instant or two before the animal actually died. At the time, I did not know what I should do with my awareness of this energy phenomenon.

Later, as a medical student, I became aware that I could perceive a similar pale yellowish hue around human patients, almost like the light thrown by a candle. The waxy light from patients reminded me of my recollections about animals. This glow would seem to shine from underneath the patient's skin. Invariably, when I saw it, patients would die soon. As their impending death drew nearer, the yellow-colored light grew more tightly focused around their bodies and faces. Watching this focusing of the light was like watching a theater spotlight drawing closer around a performer onstage.

I considered this observation to be one of my personal idiosyncrasies. For years I never felt comfortable openly sharing my personal observations with anyone but my wife, Janey. I might tell her casually in passing about a patient, "Oh, Mr. Smith is not doing well. You know, he's starting to acquire that waxy look. You know the special light." Janey would nod knowingly.

I have read and reread the works by Carlos Castaneda as many as a dozen different times. In those volumes, the Yaqui mentor, Don Juan, describes how shamans learn to see people as luminous eggs, made up of silver threads of cosmic energy that are spun into shapes and made from webs of light that reach out in all directions from the center of a person's body, near the umbilicus. Castaneda writes:

> When they are seen as fields of energy, human beings appear to be like fibers of light, like white cobwebs, very fine threads that circulate from the head to the toes. Thus to the eye of a seer, a man looks like an egg of circulating fibers. And his arms and legs are like luminous bristles, bursting out in all directions.
>
> —CARLOS CASTANEDA, *A Separate Reality*

Don Juan mentions to his apprentice Carlos that when a person is very ill and close to death, the fiber bundles retract, start to lose their luminosity, and begin to unwind. The luminous egg begins to lose its coherence and integrity. When I came upon this description in Castaneda's work, it seemed to closely match what I had observed about individuals who were near death: their luminosity seemed to move from within and then pass outward into their skin. When the luminosity reached the skin itself, it could be perceived as a pale yellowish light arising from the body itself. So maybe I was not alone in this ability to detect perceptible changes in light or energy as a person moved closer to dying.

I remember vividly the first time I saw that light coming from someone who was not a patient. One cold morning in West Roxbury, when I was a third-year medical student, I was out taking our family dog for a walk and bumped into Jim. He was the patriarch of the extended family that lived in the two-story house next to ours. I had known Jim, as a neighbor, on a casual basis for four or five years. He had always demonstrated a warm fondness for my children and all of our many dogs. Jim and I would see each other as we went about our suburban lives and our domestic chores, especially in the summer when we had barbecues to tend and lawns to mow. So it was quite natural for me to stop for a moment, as I was walking down the street, to take off my mittens and shake Jim's hand. I wanted to wish him well for the approaching Christmas holidays. As I shook Jim's hand, I immediately became aware of "the light" coming from his face. We went through some holiday pleasantries and then I asked, "Hey, Jim, how you been feelin' lately? Cold gettin' to you or anything?"

"No," he said. "I feel fit as a fiddle."

I could not forget what I had seen and I mentioned it to Janey when I got back home. "Hey, I just saw Jim while I was out walkin' the dog."

"Oh yeah? How is he?"

"Oh, fine. You know the peculiar thing is that he's got that funny waxy kind of color I tell you about that I see...the one around people who are dying."

"Oh, forget it," Janey admonished me. "It's probably just the cold changing the way his skin looks."

"Yeah, maybe. Just a little freaky, that's all."

"Well, if it will make you feel better, I'll ask his daughter, Susan, next time I see her. I'll ask how Jim's doing, okay?"

Janey was true to her word, and the next day Susan told Janey that Jim was just fine. He had just finished a routine checkup with his doctor a few months back. I did not think much about it after that. However, about two weeks after the New Year's had passed, I came home and Janey was ashen.

"What's up, honey?" I asked her with alarm.

"It's Jim. They just took him to the hospital. He started suddenly coughing up blood, and they found out he's full of lung cancer. He's in a coma and won't survive."

"Yeah, I figured. It's not like it's one hundred percent, but I'm rarely mistaken when I see that color. It almost always tells me something real bad is up."

Now, please don't get me wrong. I don't walk around the hospital evaluating the glow of people's skin and forecasting who will die. It's an epiphenomenon: maybe, as people get closer to dying, unraveling of their inner luminescence lends them a special aura. I've seen patients precariously close to dying in the ICU, who have had this soft, candle-like light come into their being. Then it faded back to a crisper, cleaner whiter light as they recovered. But when the yellowish hue comes, the individual is near death.

So this brings me to Harry Holt. I was a fourth-year medical student when Harry walked—or more precisely, rolled—into my life. I was assigned to the Cardiology Service at the Massachusetts General Hospital (MGH) under Anthony DeAngelo. Dr. DeAngelo did not have just a simple Cardiology Service; it was an empire. His patient load was so enormous that almost two floors of the hospital were devoted just to his patients. A whole separate area of the emergency room was devoted to Cardiology, because so many patients arrived at the hospital to be evaluated for chest pain or arrhythmias.

As the fourth-year student, in what was termed a "subinternship," I was supposed to act just like a resident, but with closer supervision. One of my responsibilities was to respond to any pages from the emergency room to evaluate a cardiac patient. My beeper went off and I was summoned to see a patient in bay 2 who had had a "sinker," meaning he had been found at home passed out and had some significant findings on his electrocardiogram.

I went downstairs and there was Harry Holt on a stretcher. He had the requisite oxygen mask strapped over his nose and mouth, leads on his wrists and ankles, and six lead wires pasted across his chest. Reams of EKG paper were already streaming onto the floor. Not a good sign. If his EKG had been normal, the tech would not have been running so much paper. On the monitor overhead, I could see that Harry's heart was having a tough time maintaining a reasonable rhythm. The heart would start into what is referred to as "normal sinus rhythm." It would hold that normal pace for a minute or two, and then deteriorate, becoming more erratic. It kept fluttering back and forth.

Harry was also exhibiting a few other poor prognostic signs. His blood pressure was not maintaining itself well. His EKG showed a lot of ischemic—a lack of blood flow—strain in the main pumping chamber of the heart, the left ventricle. He was sheet-white, looking like "shit split with an ax," as one resident described it. Next to Harry was standing Phyllis Holt, his wife of forty-seven years.

Despite the swarms of doctors and nurses and technicians around Harry, Phyllis was terrified. We stuck two intravenous lines into Harry and started giving him nitrates to help his oxygen-starved heart. Antiarrhythmic agents helped his myocardium get into a decent beat, to keep pumping adequately.

Phyllis mentioned to me, in our hectic introductions, that she understood arrhythmias and their dangers all too well because she had a pacemaker herself that kept her from going into complete heart block. I smiled. She smiled. I knew that she knew enough to be plenty scared for her husband.

We got Harry transferred up to the coronary care unit and kept otherwise doing that "voodoo that we do" to keep him alive. During the night, he stabilized considerably.

Phyllis told me the story of how she had been working inside their little house in Brookline and Harry had gone outside to mow the lawn. It was a hot, humid day by Boston standards, but Harry was adamant about getting the lawn done and then putting out the sprinkler.

"Harry's proud of his lawn. He likes it green. Lusher than anyone else's in the neighborhood," she added, almost apologetically. "Don't you, Harry darling?" Harry nodded sleepily.

So Phyllis had remained busy in the house and she heard the lawnmower just going and going. It seemed to just be standing still in one place for the longest time. Then the darn thing just sputtered out. After a while, Phyllis thought it funny that Harry had not returned to the house. It was more like him to come in and cool off. Or trouble her to make a lemonade or an iced tea, something sweet.

Phyllis eventually came downstairs. No sign of Harry. She went outside to admonish him to come in, and drink fluids in this kind of heat.

When she stepped outside, there was Harry face down, in the middle of the lawn. God only knew how long he had been there! She ran to turn him over and he was completely blue. She did not know which way to turn. Should she go inside and call 911? Should she try to blow some air into his mouth? She scarcely knew what to do, so she started screaming for help.

Fortunately, George, their next-door neighbor, was a fireman and was off duty. Every other weekend, he was at the station, but this was, God bless, his weekend off, so he was puttering around the house. As soon as George heard the commotion, he came running. He had his wife call an ambulance. Lord only knew, had it not been for George's presence of mind, what would have happened to Harry. Phyllis thought he would have probably died.

I nodded politely as she made her way through her story. Took an occasional note for my medical history. No, Harry had never had any cardiac problems. Yes, he had had a bit of a problem controlling his diet. He had high blood pressure. But nothing that their doctor felt that they needed to worry about. Yes, his father had died of a stroke. His younger brother, Dick, had had a heart attack two or three years ago, and had required a heart operation. But he was just fine now. The brother had even lost some weight and was playing golf now.

I told Phyllis that her husband seemed to have stabilized considerably since he had first arrived in the emergency room. It had been a very long day and she was exhausted after everything that she had been through. I encouraged her to go home to get some sleep. I took down her phone number and placed it in front of her husband's chart so everyone could find it and call her should anything change with Harry's condition. She seemed relieved that I gave her permission to go home. I reassured her that we would look after Harry and keep a close eye on things.

During the night, Harry continued to improve. His EKG revealed evidence of a fairly substantial myocardial infarction but his heart seemed to be all right. In fact, by morning, Harry was a gregarious, humorous man who seemed to be relishing just being alive, even within the drab confines of an intensive care unit.

As the "grunt" or "scut puppy" for the Cardiology Service, I had the job of going around to collect all the laboratory values, EKG strips, and physician notes, and then to write the daily progress notes for every patient in the CCU. Then the resident team gathered at 6 A.M. to go around and double-check on everything before the attending faculty came in around 8 A.M. So I went by, checked on every patient in the CCU, and had a wonderful time chatting with Harry. As one of the senior residents commented sarcastically on morning rounds to the team, "There's nothing like a near-death experience to help you prioritize your life... at least till you're better."

Harry was no different. He was overjoyed to be breathing. In fact, he was euphoric for a guy who had almost died less than twenty-four hours earlier. He was gushing with enthusiasm about "how sweet it is to just be alive."

He said to me, "Young man, take note! There's nothing that could possibly make a man feel better than to take a big deep breath and feel his heart pumping and the blood coursing through his veins!"

I thought to myself: *arteries*. You really mean blood pumping through your *arteries*, Harry old boy.

But Harry, bless his heart (so to speak), really meant it. He slapped the sides of his chest cavity with enthusiasm. It set his heart monitor off. A worried look crossed his face as the alarms starting wailing at once. A nurse came in from the outside station as I reached to turn the alarm back off.

"It's okay. It's okay. He just jiggled his leads," I yelled out to the nurse. Harry heaved a sigh of relief. "It's fine, Mr. Holt. It's just when you slap yourself that hard, it makes the EKG electrodes jump. That sends a false alarm. You're just fine." Later that morning a worried and fatigued Phyllis came to the bedside and positively smothered Harry with kisses and hugs.

A couple of days rolled along; Harry was recovering nicely. Each morning, I looked forward to stopping by his bedside and chatting with him, as I entered my daily progress note on behalf of the entire Cardiology Service and Dr. DeAngelo.

The cardiology fellows were there because of Dr. DeAngelo's reputation. They were among the best and the brightest of the nation. No one could take better care or provide more state-of-the-art care than DeAngelo's fellows. They had an international reputation to uphold. Just watching their spirit of pride and hard work was inspiring.

I grew to like Harry. In his life, he had been all over the world as a Merchant Marine. His Liberty ship had been torpedoed in the North Atlantic by U-boats and he had been one of only twenty-four sailors to be rescued from the ocean.

He carefully explained to me that when convoys were plying their way through the treacherous waters between Labrador and Ireland, the Nazis would try to cripple one of the freighters, so that the other ships in the convoy would slow down to pick up survivors. Once the ships dropped their speed, as they had to in order to take on survivors, the U-boats would close in like jackals and "blow 'em to pieces." So the convoys had developed an irrevocable policy.

"FDR, the president of the United States of America, himself had issued the order: no ship in our convoy was to cut their speed or divert from their course to help with survivors. It was understood by one and all. Every Merchant Marine knew that once they were in the drink they were on their own. Everyone accepted it even though any man would have gladly given up his life to turn around and pluck a brother out of the soup. But that was 'xactly what the krauts were hopin'. They were takin' that periscope and flippin' those crosshairs round and round, just waitin' and hopin' one ship'd cut her knots down and then kabaaam!

"The krauts were good with them fish—the torpedoes—and as soon as you'd cut her back to let's say half, or quarter speed, and then cut your rudder over to circle back, the U-boat'd be waitin'. Just where she'd need to be to bring a fish up broadside. They'd cut your ship in two. And you know, more than half the time, we'd be carrying a fair 'mount of ammunition. You know, thousands of the thirty- and fifty-millimeter rounds, hundreds of them five-pound shells. You name it, we had it aboard us as ordnance. Hell, that was our job: supplyin' the Brits and our boys with everythin' they needed for fightin'. No easy job. Well, hell, the hardest part weren't them kraut U-boats, it was watchin' a beautiful ship, half aboard was friends, blown to bits, sinkin' in front of your eyes. And...then you'd hear 'em in the water. That was rough. Leavin' 'em behind...that's the worst of it. You never forget that," Harry said, his voice trailing off.

I loved hearing about his life. After World War Two was over, Harry had worked part-time as a magician, part-time as a wholesaler for plumbing supplies. His life was a rich one. He had sailed a twenty-four-foot sailboat from Cape Cod to Key West for twelve days by himself. He had met Greta Garbo at the famous 21, as a doorman. He had shaken Ike's hand in the election campaign of 1956. He had been a limo driver in Clark Gable's funeral procession. Hell, Harry had even met Rin Tin Tin, the canine film star.

So it did not surprise Harry or me that on the fourth night after his heart attack, after he had already been transferred to a regular cardiology floor, I came by to sit down and chat with him. The myocardial infarction had filled Harry with a wonderful sense of gratitude for just being alive. He told me that he felt like he had been reborn. It was a joy for me to witness, even as a relatively young spectator who did not yet grapple well with mortality.

While I sat there (I no longer had to carry on the pretense of writing notes in his medical chart), Harry confessed to me that he had, in fact, had a near-death experience during his heart attack.

"I got to tell you that there really was nothin' scary 'bout it. I just felt at peace, loved. I just seemed to rise up in the air, like a puffy cloud. I could see myself lying in the grass. But it wasn't like I was scared or anything. I just felt like I was going home, like being on furlough to see my family during the war or something. You know, something that you're jus' dyin' to do. I suppose that's a pun or somethin'. But you get what I mean, don't you? It was like I was lookin' forward to it. Like I'd been lookin' forward to it for the longest time, and now I was goin' to finally get there, get to do it.

"Now," Harry continued, "it isn't like I wanted to die or somethin' like that. 'Cause I sure as hell didn't want to leave Phyllis. Boy, the men'd be swarmin' 'round 'er like bees 'round honey. No, siree"—he chuckled with a hint of lustful pride. "But at the same time, I knew there wasn't anything to fear 'bout what lay beyond this life." Harry got very solemn. "I jus' couldn't help but thinkin' 'bout the buddies we'd left in the sea, after them U-boats got 'em. I thought later 'bout it. I jus' kept wishin' that when the end did come for 'em that it would have been like it seemed to be for me when I had my heart attack." Tears slowly rolled down his cheeks. He was smiling at the same time. "It's like, I think, I now realize that each of 'em when they died was okay. That they are still okay now. I guess maybe it has always been okay. I just didn't know it. But it feels good to know, 'cause you can't help but wonder. Even after all these years."

The next morning when I stopped to round on Harry, things were dramatically different. Harry seemed ill at ease, like the proverbial cat on a hot tin roof, like he was uncomfortable in his own skin. I checked a rhythm strip on the EKG and drew some labs.

The worst of it was the light coming from Harry. It was that yellow, waxy light in his eyes, from his skin. I immediately transferred Harry back to the coronary care unit. That light, the sheen, made me terribly sad for Harry. I had grown to like him a lot.

The interesting thing about all this was that Harry was having no symptoms like chest pain or an arrhythmia. I had nothing solid to go on except my premonition. I told a white lie to the charge nurse to get Harry back into the CCU. I explained I thought I had seen a run of ventricular tachycardia on his monitor. I had just not been quick enough to cap-ture it on the paper strip. It had disappeared. But because ventricular tachycardia is a potentially dangerous rhythm, the supervising nurse immediately granted my request.

Harry, I believe, knew all along what was up. He never asked me once why he was heading back to the CCU. He knew. When Phyllis came, he focused on reassuring her that she had nothing to worry about. There was plenty of money in the bank. The house was paid up. I kept hovering around. Every time Harry would spook her with his talk, he would back off, reassure her, and change the topic.

Harry told Phyllis to go home, to come back in the evening. He told her he was feeling tired. He hugged her, kissed her on the lips, then kissed her on the forehead. I did not intrude but there are video cameras in every CCU room, so I could see him saying his good-byes.

After Phyllis left, I got some ominous results from the laboratory. The lab work was preliminary but suggested that Harry was about to have another myocardial infarction—a whopping tsunami of a heart attack. I went in to talk things over with Harry, but he was already holding his chest with one hand over his heart and looking up at the new bad blips showing up on the monitor. I knew. He knew.

"Harry, I've got to talk something over with you," I started.

"I know. It's a heart attack. Another one."

"Precisely, Harry. That's what the first tests seem to suggest. I need to know that it is okay with you—if we need to—to go ahead and intubate you. Put a plastic pipe down your mouth, into your windpipe, so if you have breathing problems—"

"It won't matter."

"No, come on, Harry. I've got to get permission to, for the team in case they need to proceed."

"I can give you all the permissions you want. It won't make any difference."

Harry was gripping his chest and now he was, in fact, having a run of V tach. I punched the emergency button for the nurse.

The charge nurse rushed in. "What's up?" she asked, glancing over at Harry.

"Call the code team. Get the code cart in here," I barked.

The nurse ran out. Overhead, I could hear the stat pages going out over the public address team.

Harry looked distressed. "Don't worry, kid. You can't stop to pick up stragglers. Know what I mean? Full steam ahead."

With that Harry's eyes rolled up in his head and the monitor went flat. A series of alarms went off. The code team arrived. We shocked Harry a bunch of times. We did CPR. We injected his heart with Adrenalin. Nothing we could do was going to bring him back. He was gone, back there in our wake with all his buddies from another lifetime ago.

I called Phyllis and let her know that despite everything we could do, Harry had passed away. I lied and stated that he had "slipped away peacefully." In fact, he had not really faded out as much as he burned out, like a comet. Phyllis sobbed. I don't recall her exact words, but under such circumstances, the words really don't matter. We sent a neighbor over to the house to drive her to the hospital. She sat with Harry for hours. His body cooled and stiffened. The charge nurse started pressing me to get Harry moved down to the morgue because there were two new "MIs" in the emergency room. There was never a vacant bed for long on the DeAngelo Service.

So that was the end of Harry, or so I thought. Harry was buried in a cemetery overlooking Boston Harbor. From the little hillside where his grave was located, I could see the coming and going of the tankers and freight ships and the occasional gray drab U.S. Navy vessel steaming out of the Charleston Navy Yard. I listened to the drone of the funeral service politely. As a lowly medical student, I had been dispatched as a representative from the Cardiology team. No one vital to the daily workings of the Service could be spared, so I was sent. The service ended and I remember being glad to duck back underground into the "T"—as the subway is called in Boston—and find some cool air again. The subway car rolled and clanked its way back toward the hospital.

I began once more receiving pages and dispatches from the various corners of the DeAngelo realm as soon as I returned. About five hours later, right around the beginning of the quieter hours of the evening shift, I received a call to come down to the emergency room.

I came downstairs to the "Attack Shack," as the bay was called, where the heart patients were put. The emergency team was in the full throes of a major resuscitation, residents were running around, shouting orders and slamming in more lines, while reams of EKG paper gathered around the floor like so much confetti.

I just stood by the door and when they yelled out for a lab or a request for a technician, I would pass it along.

I was surprised when the senior fellow in Cardiology called out an order for a fluoroscopy unit to be brought into the "shack." I overheard the fellow, holding up a chest X-ray to the overhead fluorescent light: "Well, Jiminy Cricket, I'll be dipped. Look at that pacemaker wire. The damned thing's broke in half."

It was only then that it dawned on me. I surged forward through the crowd to make my way to the stretcher. The Cardiology fellow was jabbing a needle about six inches long into the side of the patient's neck and looking up at the monitor till there was some wavy activity.

"There we are. Give me the leads." A nurse passed him two thin silver wires and he passed them down the needle. "Okay, battery pack! Plug her in and let's start pacing her." The nurse attached a small unit, no bigger than a cassette recorder, and turned a few knobs. Suddenly, the cardiac monitor started beeping slowly, rhythmically. The fellow sighed audibly.

"There we go. Now let's get her up to the CCU."

I looked down and saw that the patient was Phyllis.

I chickened out. I didn't have the stomach to take care of Phyllis right after Harry's death. I passed her off to another medical student. In fact, I avoided her for days and just caught snippets about her progress whenever the Cardiology residents would give reports to the other members of the team. I heard that her pacemaker wire had apparently given out and she had collapsed at Harry's grave site. There had been another burial ceremony going on, and someone had glanced up and noticed her on the ground. Someone started CPR. The rest was history.

I heard, three days later, she was going to be headed home.

"Yeah," the resident reported. "She's headed home. But she's madder than a hornet. Says she goin' to sue all our asses off for interfering with the will of God! She's asking who the hell we are to bring her back to life, when God reaches down from Heaven and cuts her pacemaker wire so she can join her husband. Don't that beat all?"

Most folks just nodded or shrugged with puzzlement. The team moved on down the hallway. Her whole saga plunged me into doubt and confusion. How were we to know what was right to do?

I still do not have a good answer to the questions posed more than twenty years ago by Phyllis and Harry. I know only two things with greater clarity now than I did then.

First, there are plenty of things worse than death. But as a culture, we have raised death to such mythical proportions that it has become more frightening and less approachable than ever before in recorded human history. I think the Egyptian culture, the Roman Empire, and even the lowliest peasant from the Middle Ages had a better handle on death than do most inhabitants of the twenty-first century. I think they would actually pity us, because now we've got so little left that most people can draw upon for any deep, abiding faith.

The second conclusion relates to Harry's so-called near-death experience. Over and over again, as I've talked with patients who've been close to death, peering into the abyss, every one of them—down to the last man or woman—has reported to me how beautifully peaceful and loving the experience of getting ready to cross over always was. Just as Harry reported, it was like coming home after being away for a long time. Most of us need to be reminded our life may begin long before, and continue long after, this singular mortal experience we are in now. We should not be crippled by the notion that only an occasional, exceptional human being achieves final spiritual transcendence beyond mortality. Instead, might we not rejoice that eternal spirit can spring forth from intermittent, mortal life experiences? That these "souls" can enrich and educate us for our personal journey?

I know that some of this may smack of elementary religious issues. Try to remember I came first with only scientific curiosity. I was not looking for any intimations beyond this mortal life. I was not a man of spiritual inclinations. I only let myself feel them when it became necessary to help me explain my own experiences. Not anyone else's.

The spiritual side of the mortal equation is not always easy to deduce. But it is a "robust" formula, balancing flesh against spirit. Stick with me. I want you to feel the spiritual echoes, as they resonated through my own experiences with patients, not as cognitive or theological arguments but as visceral installments.

Four

Is There a Doctor in the House?

When I graduated from Harvard Medical School in 1982, I had 114 fellow students getting their M.D. degrees with me. I have seen lots of graduations in my life, but nothing came close to the grandeur and pomp that we all experienced that May morning, gathered with our families, on the medical school's quadrangle, with its commanding expanse spilling onto Longwood Avenue.

The class of '82 had chosen Professor Judah Folkman as its convocation speaker. Dr. Folkman was one of the finest teachers and inspirational figures who have ever graced the halls of the medical school. He was one of the youngest people ever named to be the chief of Pediatric Surgery at Boston's Children's Hospital. Even more interesting, though, was the fact that Dr. Folkman would, in fact, later step down from his position as the head of Surgery to take a much less prestigious position as a simple researcher, because he believed that he could make a more important contribution as a researcher than as a surgeon. He stepped out of the limelight for something in which he believed. To be a surgeon, any surgeon, requires an ego. There's an old joke among surgeons: A surgeon is asked who he thinks might be the three greatest surgeons in the world. He always has trouble coming up with two other names besides his own. It took a lot of *cajones* for Dr. Folkman to give up being surgeon in chief.

In fact, he did make the right decision. Dr. Folkman later went on to define an entirely new scientific field of tumor angiogenesis, related to how a tumor survives and grows by recruiting blood supply. He argued, correctly, that no one has ever died from a small, insignificant cancer. It's massive, infiltrating, seeding tumors that are reaching out everywhere, gobbling every tissue and organ in sight, that kill people. He hypothesized that if one learned to keep tumors from ever growing big, one could effectively control cancerous growth and stop malignant tumors from killing people. His seemingly simple idea revolutionized the way folks think about therapeutic approaches in oncology. His theory proved to be absolutely correct. He was even nominated for the Nobel Prize in medicine. His answer to the news that he might be awarded the greatest prize in all of medicine? He was too busy in the lab to have his photograph taken. Dr. Folkman hates publicity. I've come to the conclusion that real heroes always do.

So as the graduating Harvard Medical School seniors, we were a bit taken aback when Professor Folkman announced that he wanted to give a convocation speech entitled "Is There a Doctor in the House?" We thought the answer was obvious: Of course there's a doctor in the house! There were, in fact, 114 new doctors in the house, graduating that very day under his nose.

What Dr. Folkman was trying to point out was that merely having a medical degree behind our names did not make us doctors. He had something else in mind.

He explained in his speech that these days patients were plagued by far too many physicians and too few doctors. Specialists for the left lung and another for the right kidney. An expert in maladies of the big toe, or the left cornea. But where was the doctor? The one who said to the patient, "I'm here for you. I'll insist that all the consulting specialists go through me. I'll ensure that every morning and every evening there is someone you can identify as *your* doctor."

Dr. Folkman was not talking about just any doctor in his commencement speech. He meant *the* doctor. He meant the physician in whom you put your trust and your life. So as we looked at one another in bewilderment on that quadrangle, we wondered who among us would become doctors and who among would remain M.D.s—technicians only.

Never was this more clearly demonstrated for me than when I was rounding with Eliot Salkner on the Cardiology Service at the Brigham and Women's Hospital in Boston. Professor Salkner was another illustrious cardiologist of the twentieth century. He was what I would call a great doctor. Maybe not always such a good one. He had written over a dozen textbooks and had more than two hundred Cardiology fellows who had trained under him. At the time, what Dr. Salkner didn't know about cardiology was probably not worth learning. Even Dr. DeAngelo at the rival Massachusetts General Hospital would admit that.

Even if you could not tell that Professor Salkner was an important man just by his demeanor, you would know it once you saw him whirling around on the various floors of the hospital, surrounded by a cloud of fawning attendings, fellows, senior residents, junior residents, interns, visiting scholars, charitable donors, and lowly medical students.

There was an elderly patient, Guiseppe Giovanni, on Dr. Salkner's service, who had a huge heart murmur, a kind of "blowing" sound you heard when you listened to his chest with a stethoscope. It sounded like the great exhalation of a breaching whale. But this sound occurred after every single beat of his heart. That murmur told us Mr. Giovanni's aortic valve was narrowed, and that every time his left ventricle contracted, it had to push a beat's worth of blood through a narrow, high-resistance circuit. Eventually, the left ventricle would just poop out under the load imposed by the constricted outlet. The solution was a new aortic valve. At the time, most aortic replacement valves were harvested from pigs. Mr. Giovanni simply could not believe his ears when Dr. Salkner came into his room to recommend that Mr. Giovanni let himself be put under anesthesia so his God-given valve could be removed and a *porcine* valve put in its place.

"A porcelain valve? Why would you want to put in a porcelain valve? Isn't it going to break? Like a teacup?" he asked.

"Mr. Guiseppe—" Dr. Salkner began.

"Giovanni. It's Giovanni."

"Mr. Giovanni. I said *porcine*. Porcine! Not *porcelain!* Porcine! Made from pigs. Well, the valve comes from a pig. A pig's heart."

That was even more distressing to Mr. Giovanni. "A pig. Maria! Why would you put pieces from a pig inside of me?"

"Well," Dr. Salkner explained, "if we don't, you will die. You will undoubtedly die from end-stage congestive failure of the left ventricle." The Cardiology fellows all murmured in agreement. "I have seen your angiogram, Mr. Giovanni. It is not pretty. No, not at all. I would say that you might have as little as a few weeks to live unless we proceed with surgery. Of that much, sir, I am certain!"

Mr. Giovanni went pale at the pronouncement. "A few weeks?"

"If that."

"Oh, my. I had no idea it was that bad, doctor."

"Well, I'm afraid it is. So I have recommended that you undergo surgery without delay. I have asked Dr. Steiner, one of our finest cardiac surgeons, to operate on you in the morning."

"Well, I'm not sure. A pig valve? That's what you want me to do? Tomorrow? Well, I'm…I'm not sure. I've got to talk to my children, to discuss this with…and my doctor. I've gotta ask my doctor's opinion."

"Your doctor?"

"Yes, my doctor."

"Well, I can assure you, sir, that I will be happy to explain the findings on your angiogram to your physician. I can tell you that he will concur with my opinion." You could tell that Professor Salkner knew no one would dare disagree with a "Salkner diagnosis."

"Well, I want my doctor's opinion."

"Sir, give me his name and phone number—"

"You don't need to call him," said Mr. Giovanni.

"Well, I thought it might help if he heard it straight from my mouth—in case he had any questions."

"Well," Mr. Giovanni said, "you can just ask him now. He's standing right there at the back of the room." Everyone audibly gasped. Who could this person be? A Cardiology fellow? A visiting doctor from the community?

The crowd of white coats parted. And there, standing in the doorway, was none other than a lowly third-year medical student.

"There!" shouted Mr. Giovanni. "There, that's my doctor! He takes care of me every day. Sees me every morning. You ask him if he approves, and then I'll sign whatever papers you want."

It was amazing to see Dr. Salkner puff himself up and then get deflated by a medical student. But that was precisely who Mr. Giovanni identified as his doctor. To Dr. Salkner's credit, he took a deep breath, scowled at his own fellows, then stepped up to the medical student and patiently explained the findings. He asked the medical student if he "wouldn't mind sitting down with his patient, Mr. Giovanni, and reassuring him of the clinical wisdom in proceeding with a porcine aortic valve replacement before there was irreparable damage to the left ventricle." When Mr. Giovanni was content with proceeding with surgery, Professor Salkner would be happy to ask Professor Steiner to see the patient and prepare him for surgery. The medical student nodded his assent and stood next to Mr. Giovanni's bed. The rest of the team swept out of the room and on to the next patient. The medical student pulled up a chair, sat down next to Mr. Giovanni, patted his hand, and started to carefully explain about aortic valves and replacement parts from pigs.

Mr. Giovanni sailed through the surgery and returned to his flat in Boston's North End. He had found his "doctor in the house." There's always one there. They're just not easy to find.

But that is what patients are looking for. In this day of innumerable lawsuits, the main issues for the plaintiffs (the patients) always seem to come down to a lack of communication between patient and physician. On daily rounds in the hospital, I am struck how many patients do not know who their attending physician is, who the doctor is who is ultimately in charge of their care. I'll hear things like "I'm on the Trauma

Service and they're the doctors who write my orders." Or I'll ask a question like "Who performed your surgical procedure on you?" Often the patient will answer something like: "I don't know exactly. There was a resident who came out and talked to my family but that may not be the one who did the surgery. I don't think it was, at least." Or more devastating perhaps, sometimes the patient will confess that he's never met his attending but he hopes to meet him before getting discharged so he can say "thank you." Or you'll hear, "I don't know who my doctor is. There's a whole bunch of them. But maybe you can ask the nurse and she'll know who you need to call."

When I first started out, as an attending, I had this crazy notion that I was too busy to see every single patient that belonged to me. I was in such a hurry, so busy operating at full speed (and, frankly, so interested in generating surplus bonus revenues), that I had somehow convinced myself it was appropriate for me to focus my efforts exclusively on those patients who were sick or had a difficult postoperative course. What was the point of stopping by to see a patient who was doing perfectly well?

You might ask how I would know if patients were doing well or not if I didn't look in on them. Good question. My reasoning—reflective of my training—was that residents were out there to do just that. They were like the DEW—distant early warning—radar system for patient care. I convinced myself that with my "drones" out seeing the patients in the floor, I would be duly notified when someone required my attention. But that begs the bigger question, I guess: Was I really their doctor? Of course, I would have flunked that test. I had a responsibility for anyone who was my patient, but could I learn to see it as more than that? More than duty? More a question of compassion? Something I wanted to do because it felt right?

My aversion to the military eventually underwent a dramatic change—a reversal. I joined the U.S. Army Medical Corps as a reservist. I had been attracted by the possibility of using the extra monies from my reserve duties to start paying off my student loans from medical school. But more enticing for me was the prospect of getting commissioned and paid by the army to help carry out research on new pharmacologic agents to protect troops from the crippling effects of low oxygen on the central nervous system when deployed to high altitude.

As a young adult I had developed a passion for mountaineering. The Alps, the Rockies, the Tetons—I would climb anywhere, anytime. Joining the army now provided me with an opportunity to combine my love of climbing with my research interests in brain function. I got to mingle with the elite of the climbing world, men and women who had been to the highest peaks on Earth. In the Army Medical Corps, I also had unlimited access to the largest, most sophisticated high-altitude chamber in the world for any of my research projects.

In 1988, the army even asked me to lead a twenty-man medical research expedition of elite soldiers and scientists to Alaska. For six weeks we studied the effects of high-altitude acclimatization on dozens of climbing teams as they struggled to make the final push to the summit of the highest mountain in North America: Mount McKinley. This massive mountain lies close to the Arctic Circle and rises to 20,333 feet above sea level. For a month and a half, during the peak climbing season, we maintained a full research camp at 16,000 feet. Many days the temperature reached 30 below zero. Not only did our party carry out scientific research, we also launched more than twenty rescue missions to save climbers who had become hurt or stranded on the dangerous slopes of the mountain. We were even able to summit the great peak ourselves after seven different attempts that had been turned back by weather or rescue priorities.

On the day we were scheduled to finally break camp and get off the mountain to hot showers and real beds, our team was called back to rescue a Korean climber stuck on the west wall of McKinley—a treacherous, dangerous expanse of snow, ice, and rock. The injured climber could not move, and we could not climb up safely to where he lay. We ordered a CH-47 Chinook helicopter from Fort Wainwright and, along with two very brave pilots, successfully carried out what was then a world's record for the highest helicopter rescue, at over 19,000 feet—far beyond the manufacturer's specs for the helicopter. We could only pray that the maxed-out jet engines could hold us in a hover, despite the dangerously thin air, while our medical team was lowered to save the stricken climber. The mission was a gratifying success. It was also the privilege of a lifetime to lead such dedicated men and women.

The research we carried out in 1988 on the mountain in Alaska paved the way for two new medications that protected troops who needed to be rapidly inserted at high altitudes. These drugs allowed us to put our Special Forces into the mountains of Pakistan and Afghanistan after 9/11 without high-altitude cerebral edema claiming a single American's life—something of which I am very proud to have been a part.

So I loved the opportunities the army offered in altitude research. But the reserves have a specific military purpose—to be ready for war. And no sooner had I bought a new home, moved my young family to Tucson, and taken up my faculty position as assistant professor of neurosurgery at the University of Arizona than I was called up in late 1990 to active duty to serve as a surgeon in Operation Desert Storm—the first of America's wars in the Gulf region of the Middle East.

During active duty, I suffered a severe back injury after a terrible fall. I was eventually transported to a hospital bed back in Fort Sam Houston, Texas. An important decision would have to be made about whether to operate on the fractures discovered in my back. I was confined to complete bed rest. I found myself waiting on pins and needles every day for my surgical team to round on me and give me some information—any information—on how I was doing, on what might be happening to me. It occurred to me that I was waiting all day long to spend thirty to forty-five precious seconds with "my team" of doctors. It was the high point of the day—the focus of my entire existence in that hospital bed. I wanted to hear the results of my latest X-ray studies or medication changes. Later, in the evening, the nurse would patiently hold the phone to my ear as I repeated every word to my wife back in Tucson.

I was just like any other patient, waiting for my doctor. What if my doctor decided I was recovering nicely and I really did not need a visit that day? How could I have been so blind to what my own patients were experiencing?

If I recovered, I swore, I would round on every patient of mine I had, without exception. All the way through residency, I thought it was about efficiency, speed, and accuracy, when it was really about compassion. How had I finished residency training for eight years and missed such a fundamental premise of patient care? In the convocation speech, that was what Dr. Folkman had been trying to point out. That it was possible for a doctor to finish, to even succeed at residency training, and miss the critical aspects of being a doctor to one's patients. Maybe my failure to see it for so long suggests a great gap in my own character. Perhaps. But it took that seminal experience of lying in a hospital bed as a patient for me to complete that critical part of my education.

I was fortunate to recover ultimately from my spine injury. But I had to learn to use my legs again, how to walk. I set myself the goal of first getting to the end of my driveway—a distance of less than thirty feet. Eventually I was able to walk my kids to the bus stop, more than a block and a half away. After standing every day for weeks with the usual moms waiting for the bus, I began to clearly see the world of my children's friends and schoolmates emerging for the first time. I began to learn names. First, those of close friends. Then brothers and sisters. Later, even their dogs, cats, and guinea pigs. I realized my whole world had collapsed around my single-minded ambition to become a neurosurgeon. I had passed up a lot of my children's lives. I desperately wanted to change my priorities, as a father and as a physician.

Six months later, I walked back into University Medical Center convinced that if I became a better man, a better husband, and a better father, then I would actually turn into a better physician too. What Dr. Folkman was trying to warn us about in that convocation speech was that the wisdom and insight a physician can acquire is dictated not by what we learn in medical school but from life experience, our own and those of our patients.

Five

No One Dies with Harvard Numbers

Some people hear their inner voice with great clarity and they live by what
they hear. They become crazy but they become legends.
One Stab, from the movie *Legends of the Fall*

Street life is hard in Boston, murderous in the winter as the outside temperatures plunge into single digits. When a nor'easter, known locally as "the Montreal Express," blows through, there's an icy cold culling. In one bad winter storm in the mid-1980s, twenty-one homeless people froze to death in a single night. Every police cruiser, tow truck, and off-duty cab was put into service to roam the city in an attempt to rescue anyone who had not already succumbed to the cold.

At the time, I was serving as the lowly surgical intern on the "Red Service" at the MGH. We saw a huge volume of indigent, homeless street people. I'm not proud to say it, but we referred to these street people collectively as "dirtballs." These were the folks you stepped over, physically and psychically, as you walked down the street.

Silvio Bustamante was one of the legendary dirtballs. He had been on the streets for over twenty years. He was a legend within the hospital. Every resident who worked there knew Silvio—nicknamed "Rocky." His medical chart ran for seven volumes; he had contracted practically every disease known to mankind: tuberculosis, hepatitis, pancreatitis, pneumonia, sepsis, and open, maggot-infested sores—not to mention, stab wounds. He'd been treated for gonorrhea more than two dozen times, which was something of a record in the annals of the hospital; hence, his nickname: Rocky—the Italian Stallion.

Rocky was pushing sixty-five (close to a hundred in street years). No homeless person stayed alive that long. But he was also coming to the end of his game. When he came in, it was always with something bad, a medical crisis that consumed every waking moment of a resident's time. Just summarizing his medical history from the chart could keep an intern up half the night.

No resident wanted Rocky on his surgical service. It was like the kiss of death. Every organ system in his body had been hammered. He had only one kidney; his liver couldn't make enough protein to provide circulating coagulation factors. Every bone in his body had been broken either from falling down while drunk, being hit by a car while drunk, or being mugged while drunk. He had gone into renal failure a half-dozen times. His immune system had given up the ghost a long while back.

Rocky should have died, by all rights, years before, but he was like the proverbial Timex watch, which "takes a licking and keeps on ticking." He was like a cat with nine lives. Somehow the docs in the hospital always put him back together. His organs hung on in precarious harmony till the next calamity struck. So during the bad winter in my internship year, the police rounded up as many dirtballs as they could before they froze. Rocky was brought in and dumped in our Emergency Department. My heart sank. He was going to be all mine. I knew it'd be awful.

I could smell Rocky halfway down the hall. I saw the nurses coming out of his room wearing surgical masks. The masks weren't for fighting off infection. When someone smelled so bad that you couldn't stand it without retching, you poured essence of orange oil on a sponge and stuck it on the inside of a surgical mask, overwhelming any other smells. Rocky's stench was an overpowering cross between rot and puke.

This time he was not only frozen like a giant Popsicle from the storm, he was vomiting up enormous gobs of clotted blood. Some as big as melons. As bad as it was to smell, it was worse to watch. Rocky was still half drunk and half hypothermic, and completely crazed. He was hallucinating but I could tell he was also in excruciating pain. He would wrap his wiry arms around his right leg. It was frozen black and already gangrenous. Between yells of agony and screeches of terror, he would suddenly stop all sound. He'd turn dark blue, then gray, and vomit a red eruption. Geysers of blood ran down the walls and the sides of the bed. It splattered on the floor. A scene of greater misery was hard to imagine. Rocky looked like a character drawn from biblical damnation. As bad as he smelled, there was no way my heart could remain unmoved by his suffering.

We put in large-bore intravenous lines. I did enough lab tests to keep the technicians up half the night. I called the blood bank and started transfusing him, not only with packed red cells but also with plasma to correct the imbalance in his clotting factors. Until this enormous bleeding problem was under control, I couldn't even schedule the necessary amputation of his right leg.

By morning, Rocky had "Harvard numbers"—his blood indices, electrolytes, liver chemistries, and renal function were all tuned back into normal range. We had an expression that went, "No one can die if they have Harvard numbers." Meaning if you got all the patient's physiological functions dialed in perfectly, there's simply nothing to die from. I had passed an endoscope down him during the night and found several varices—enlarged veins—at the base of his esophagus that were bleeding, and I managed somehow to electrically coagulate them. Then we had to trim his dead leg off just below the knee. It took less than an hour.

How was he going to fare—this old, lone wolf of the North End—as a peg leg? Every day his body tried to somehow rebel against my insistent ministrations. He went into alcohol withdrawal and developed delirium tremens (DTs) and seizures. When I got that under control, he developed a urinary tract infection that threatened to go after his single, worn-out kidney. When I smothered that fire with antibiotics, he vomited, and sucked half of his dinner into his lungs and then developed a terrible pneumonia that kept him on a ventilator for a week. Since he could not eat, I had to put a feeding tube in his stomach to keep him alive. Managing Rocky was like herding a bunch of crazed physiological cats, determined to scatter his body's functions in every direction.

For eight straight weeks, I took care of him—every single blip in his blood chemistries, every shadow on his X-rays, every ounce of fluid that moved in or out of him was mine to watch over. The burden of Rocky was on my shoulders. Everyone on the team knew it. Secretly they relished it. Every resident had been through at least one bout with him. It was a matter of pride for all of us. They knew I was struggling, but I kept on going. Our reputation as the Red Service depended on keeping him alive. After all, a dozen teams at the hospital had done it before us. We weren't going down in history as the team that let Rocky die on our watch. Not us.

In retrospect, the way we talked and thought about our patients seems shameful. But we were more like soldiers at the front than doctors. Suffering and death narrowed our vision. We were locked in a battle of wits and guts, fighting desperately to keep people alive. There wasn't anything else to feel.

Eventually, Rocky's body responded to my relentless care. He was out of the ICU, dried out, and off booze for the time being. His blood counts came back reasonably well, especially in light of his inherently fragile body. The amputated stump below his knee was healing. On rounds, I had fewer fires to put out. Each morning, as the data at his bedside became increasingly optimistic, we congratulated ourselves for upholding the standards of the Red Service!

It was clear that we had to "place" Rocky somewhere. We couldn't send him limping back into the Boston winter. We'd have to "turf him"—meaning we would have to find a rehabilitation unit or nursing home that would take him. That was a daunting task. Almost every health care institution within a hundred-mile radius of the hospital had heard about Rocky by reputation. No one was going to take him without a fight. Rocky was a handful even when he was relatively healthy and sober. There was always the drink. Sooner or later, he'd get some. Then he'd career into some new health crisis, usually a very expensive one for whatever facility had accepted him.

Turfing Rocky was going to be one of my crowning achievements as an intern. As he got stronger on his first prosthesis, he started walking (and falling) in every hallway and threshold in the hospital. I'd have to steer this pariah of a patient to some new, distant shore. I spent hours on the phone. Finally I found a rehab hospital in town, with a new wing, that had just opened. Here was my chance! Too new to know anything yet about the legendary Rocky.

When I announced the news on morning rounds, there were cheers (as I said earlier, sensitivity wasn't one of our strengths) from the team. Rocky looked up in puzzlement. He just uttered, "I won't be going to any rehab."

He hadn't said more than a dozen words during his entire hospital admission, not counting when he was screaming about the spiders on the walls in the throes of the DTs. Otherwise, it was pretty much limited to "Mornin', doc." So I was shocked at his reaction, but I decided he was just being a stubborn jerk. In my opinion, there was no reason he should care.

"Listen to me, Rocky," I said. "You've got to go to rehab to get that leg of yours working, so you can get around without crutches."

"Nope, I won't go. I'm going to go be with my son," he said in a matter-of-fact way.

His son? We didn't know anything about a family. This changed everything. Now we had a relative to work with.

The senior resident intervened. "Don't you worry, Rocky, we'll have Dr. Hamilton swing by later and work out arrangements with your son." He winked at me. My mind was racing. Why had I been killing myself all this time to place him when there was family who could assume responsibility for him?

The rest of the team was all smiles. Rocky was as good as gone. Or in intern jargon, "AMF." Let's just say that stands for "Adios, my friend."

Again, I'm not sharing these tidbits because I'm proud of them. But I have a sense of belonging to an elite group of the surgeons training at MGH. We used to muse that the abbreviation MGH stood for "Man's

Greatest Hospital." But we were not immune to human suffering, so we developed verbal armor—often hard, sarcastic defenses. Sometimes fatalistic. Usually arrogant.

After rounds, I practically bounced over to Rocky's bed. I was overjoyed. He had a son! He was going to Spaulding Rehabilitation Hospital. I needed a phone number. Let the son know. Maybe he could even drive Rocky over? I sat on the edge of the bed. It was the first time I'd ever sat down to talk to Rocky. I'd probed every orifice in his body and stuck a needle into almost every organ, but I'd never sat on his bed. I didn't ask his permission (I should have) and landed on his stump by accident.

"You sat on my stump, bozo," he said.

"Sorry, Rocky." I jumped back up. As I began to explain his rehab transfer, his face darkened with anger.

"Listen, I already told you! I'm not going anywhere, except to see my son, got it?"

"Well, yes, of course." I began blabbering. "You know, Rocky, this is the first that I'm hearing about your son. I didn't know you had family around...."

"You never asked," he said bluntly.

That was true. We'd all assumed there was no one. Street people didn't have families, did they?

I offered to call Rocky's son. He said no. I explained there were arrangements to work out.

"Let me phone him," I pleaded.

"Nope, you can't," he insisted.

"I can't?" I was getting steamed. "Why can't I?"

"Because he's dead. That's why!"

Was he being sarcastic? I knew he was angry.

"I see.... You mean he's..."

"I mean he's dead," he said flatly. "Just dead."

I shut up. This wasn't what it seemed. Maybe Rocky was hallucinating. The situation required some finesse on my part. I sat down again, this time with attention as to where.

"Rocky, tell me about your son," I said.

At first he was reluctant. But things had been bottled up far too long. Apparently, his boy had been a great kid. A good ballplayer. People used to joke he should join the Red Sox. As Rocky talked, he got a faraway look.

"My kid didn't want to be a ballplayer," Rocky said. "He wanted to be a lawyer. Just like the one Spencer Tracy played in *Inherit the Wind*. He said one day he wanted to argue a case in front of the Supreme Court."

Then he said, "I guess he wanted to follow in his old man's footsteps." Tears welled up in his eyes.

"You were an attorney?" I asked incredulously.

"Yeah. Hard to believe. But it's true. Made partner before I was thirty," Rocky said with a note of satisfaction. "I was a golden boy, back in the forties, right after World War Two. Partner. Everything."

Could he be making the whole thing up? No. There was an intensity and solemnity in his voice. He was speaking the truth.

"I was a hot litigator once," Rocky continued. "I had everything. A house in Back Bay. A summer place in Wellfleet Harbor. Even a forty-five-foot yacht. Called her the *Scrimshaw Queen*. She was a sleek double-master. Jackie was a good sailor too. He could outtack, outsail anyone. Great navigator too."

"So what happened?" I asked.

"You mean how did a top lawyer end up a dirtball?"

I winced at the term. I didn't think patients ever heard our degrading nicknames for them.

He took a deep breath and held it. It tightened his whole frame. He drew himself up.

"Jackie went to Harvard Law. That's what happened. And a year and a half into it, he took a leave of absence to go to Vietnam. Joined the Marine Corps and became a fighter pilot. That was my Jackie."

"And what happened?"

Rocky's face distorted. "Some..." He started to cry. "Shot down. Ground-to-air missile... My boy...!"

He couldn't go on.

He wept for five minutes. Eventually he lifted his head and grabbed a towel.

"Hey, I am sorry," he said as he collected himself.

"Please, don't worry about it," I answered.

"Well, when Jackie died, I fell apart. Nothing mattered. Not the law firm. Not my marriage. I was glad to find the bottle, truth be told. It's not like the booze saved me, but it filled the hole, you know? Booze can do that."

"So what do you mean you're going to go see him?" I prodded gently.

"Well, Jackie came to see me last night in a dream, and he told me we were going to be together."

I was concerned about how Rocky was thinking. "Go on," I said.

"That's it. I may be a drunk, but I'm stone-cold sober right now. You know it. Just like you're here right now. Jackie came to see me last night and swore we'd be together again. Once and for all." He smiled. There was a solemn formality in his words.

I didn't know how to respond. But I had enough sense to excuse myself. I double-checked his chart. Yep. Still Harvard numbers.

Rocky's numbers were perfect. I went back to his bedside. He was as lucid as I was. But we still had to get him to rehab. That was the mission.

"Rocky, I understand your boy's coming to see you. In your dream. I still have to make some arrangements so we can get you transferred to Spaulding, okay?"

I offered to get him a haircut and a shave, to spiff him up a bit.

At that time, the hospital had a full-time barber and hairdresser on staff. They usually tended to the well-heeled patients. Nothing elevates a patient's spirits more than a good shave. A trim. Getting the hair done. It's a pity these days, in our rush to cut health care costs, we've eliminated so many personal touches and services.

I called Elwood, the hospital barber, and asked him to come over and get Rocky looking sharp. Elwood was as kind a person as you'd ever find and sometimes did haircuts for nothing. Rocky looked like a Neanderthal out of one of those prehistoric dioramas at the Natural History Museum. His gray hair was disheveled and hung down to his shoulders. His beard was just as long. Elwood would have to work his magic on this one.

In the meantime, I made arrangements for an ambulance to take Rocky to rehab. I knew I was betraying him. It had to be done. Even if I'd wanted to, there was no way we could keep Rocky in the hospital. It was too costly.

I went back to see Elwood's handiwork. It was miraculous. Rocky was all trimmed. The beard was gone. He looked a bit like that high-priced lawyer he had been in the past. He'd been a handsome man. With a square jaw and a strong face. His nose was askew because it had been broken many times in fights and beatings. But now I had a glimpse of the man he had once been.

The nurses came in. They fussed over him, commenting on how hand-some he looked. He smiled, bathing in their compliments. Losing his son cast him in a whole new light. He was no longer a dirtball—maybe he was even a bit of a hero. Then the ambulance came. I looked at Rocky. He looked back at me. He seethed with resentment. I felt like Judas.

"I told you I'm going to see Jackie. You knew that," he said, as they took him out the door. I stared after him. But I also felt relief. After eight weeks of continuous medical care and attention, he was finally gone. I was free. And I felt victorious too.

I returned to the dozens of patients on the Red Service, burying myself in the endless day of an intern. My mind was already absorbed with other concerns. An hour later came the stat page to an outside line. The medical director at Spaulding was on the line. He was furious.

"I'm reporting you to Dr. Austen, the head of Surgery!" he screamed into the phone. "You should be ashamed of yourself, sending us a patient in Mr. Bustamante's condition!"

"What condition? What's wrong with him?" I was incredulous.

"What's wrong? Hell, they rolled him in the door here and he began exsanguinating in the lobby. Just started vomiting. I don't have to tell you what a shock it was to our staff and our visitors! We just opened a few days ago. No one was prepared for this kind of a disaster!"

Rocky must have popped another venous varix in his esophagus.

Maybe Harvard numbers couldn't protect against every mishap.

"Well, I'm sorry. We treated the esophageal varices. He hadn't bled in eight weeks. Just send him back. We'll take care of it," I suggested.

"Well, Dr. Hamilton, we can't do that. He died in the lobby. Not five minutes ago!"

"No," I whispered.

He could tell I was in shock. His tone softened.

"I'm sorry. The bleeding was so extensive, so sudden. It just happened."

"I know." And I knew Rocky was gone. With his Jackie. Harvard numbers couldn't stop it.

Early in our surgical career, we throw ourselves against the obstacles embodied in our patients. We see, as I did in Rocky's case, the patients' ailments and diseases set forth like enemies, massing against us. You attack each one, sharpening your sword to slay them, stabbing away until you get the right answer. Till you defeat them. Naturally, if you frame each disease in such a context, you'll come to see the patient as little more than a kind of vessel—the body into which the problem has been poured. Later, it dawns on you that the patients need to be more than just problems waiting for elegant solutions.

One of the great secrets of medicine is that, as a physician, you have unparalleled entry into the lives of others. Every patient is an existential conduit to seeing your own struggles. Each patient brings you one step closer to seeing the truth about yourself. At the time, I knew that Rocky's dream of rejoining his son was a vision meant to bring closure to his life. I could not concede that Rocky could succumb on my service, on my watch. That losing him was not a defeat.

Six

From Flesh to Spirit

Life cannot wait until the sciences may have explained the universe scientifically.
We cannot put off living until we are ready.

JOSÉ ORTEGA Y GASSET

I n each of our lives occur transformational moments, fragile as spun glass. They drift through our lives for a fraction of a second and then shatter. There's no guarantee we will be able to visualize these critical instants when they burst into existence. To do so, we must learn to gaze obliquely at their evanescent scope and beauty. We'll see lives of those we love, of strangers, of animals, trees, mountains, and seas—all woven into one intimate and continuous network of life stretching across all manner of time and space.

I want to be clear with you about these revelations. This feeling— I don't want you to misunderstand when I say that a person just *feels* these delicate moments—you don't just *feel* them. They hit you. Like a fist. There's nothing delicate about the awakening these moments trigger. Certainly not this one moment in 1982. About halfway through the first year of internship, on my printed schedule was a two-month stint on the Burn Service. As soon as internship began, I'd learned all residents dreaded this assignment. Something about the Burn Rotation gave everyone the creeps. I had no idea what everyone was so afraid of. Since we'd already seen every permutation on the theme of human suffering and disfigurement, what could be left?

There are two parts to the Burn Service. One place you could end up was Bigelow 13. While most architects and building engineers avoid the designation of a thirteenth floor because of latent superstition, whoever built the Bigelow Building at MGH had no such concerns. Bigelow 13, as luck would have it, was the Adult Burn Service ward. As you emerged from the elevators, an archway led you onto the A ward. The arch was painted dazzlingly white. In exquisitely drawn Gothic letters, were the words "Welcome to Bigelow 13—A Great Place to Visit." Bigelow 13 was considered the choice assignment, the lesser of two evils on the Burn Service. There was far worse: the Shrine.

The Shriners Burn Institute is a dark, monolithic building, rising starkly. It stood alone, separate from the rest of the hospital campus. The six-story structure was built through the contributions of thousands of devoted Shriners, a philanthropic and social organization that is derived from the Freemasons and has now built a network of over twenty pediatric hospitals, open to any child free of charge. Since its opening, the Shrine (as it was known) had served as the major center for almost every pediatric burn victim along most of the eastern seaboard. The surgical residents nicknamed it Crispy Critters. The Pediatric Burn Center at the Shrine was the closest thing any of the residents could conjure up as Hell on Earth. There, dozens of mutilated, suffering children were huddled into one somber, sorrowful building. Most residents never talked openly about Crispy Critters. That residents are given to derogatory labels is a measure of how horrifying these places really are to us. Just as on the battlefield—where monikers emerge like "Pork Chop Hill," "Massacre Mile," and "Dead Man's Ditch"—we have to be able to put names to these places, a spot on the map of human tragedy.

My first day there, the head nurse took me around. She must have known from experience how scared all the new surgical residents were of the burned children. She seemed intent on focusing my attention on the auditorium, the Xerox machine, the fridge, even the video game stations, where the residents played after the children were asleep. But eventually the time came to finally see *them*. Before going onto the unit, we had to don sterile scrub suits with hoods and put masks over our faces. The nurse told me we would be seeing the big burns—"the eighty-percenters or higher."

As the translucent glass doors hissed apart, we entered into an alien world—an encampment. The room was bathed in the purple glow of ultraviolet lights, aimed at reducing bacterial counts in the air. Each child was surrounded by huge plastic drapes, walling out the bacteria that were stalking them. There were large sterile ports in the sides of each veil, where nurses could insert their arms to change dressings, plug in IVs, or give injections.

Devices made whining, sucking, and bubbling noises. A robotic chorus rising up around each child's buried, pupal form. Each child was like a mummy, wrapped in bandages. Goggles were placed over the eyes. There were no openings for air. Here and there, a tube or line broke through the weave of the dressing, delivering or evacuating across the white gauze landscape. Only the familiar shape, outlined by dressings, hinted that human children might lie buried below. Were it not for the frenzied activity of the machines, there was nothing to suggest the larval forms were even alive.

I worked hard to admire all the sophisticated equipment and precautions assembled to protect sterility. It sent a shiver through me. Here, the technical mastery of asepsis had risen to the level of absurd wizardry.

Only the nurse's cheerful voice sustained me.

"And over here," she said, as she made a graceful arm movement, "is Joey!"

I looked. Another nondescript mummy.

"Joey and his friend found a fifty-gallon drum of gasoline and tried to set it on fire," she explained. "But it exploded. Of course. Killed the other boy, Joey's friend. What was his name? Let's see.... Bertram. Bertram was the one killed."

I figured Bertram was the luckier of the two.

"Joey received a ninety-five-percent burn," she continued in a monotonous nasal twang. "He lost his ears. He also lost fingers, toes. His nose was burned. His eyelids gone. He only has a few small patches of skin left. There's one small patch inside each armpit. Of course, there's also a small patch in the groin. Those were spared."

"Of course," I gulped in horror. There was a pair of goggles on Joey's mummied head. "Can he close his eyes?" I asked, wondering if that might be the reason for the goggles.

"Oh, no. He can't. No eyelids, as I said. Besides, his corneas were scorched."

I felt sick to my stomach. "Well, what are the goggles for, then?" I asked, struggling not to vomit. "He's blind. Why does he need goggles?"

"I suppose they protect his eyes for some reason."

I had never seen so much suffering concentrated in one place. How would I get through this rotation? It seemed unendurable.

We left the ICU, known affectionately as "Mummy World," and crossed over into what was called "Camp Chronic." Camp Chronic was the ward floor where the survivors from Mummy World eventually arrived for endless rounds of reconstructive surgery. After a while on the Burn Service, one realized that Camp Chronic was more than a hospital ward. It was a human laboratory.

Here the children became living "clay" where generations of surgeons (myself included) practiced and perfected reconstructive surgical techniques. Each generation created more brilliant restorative landscapes out of the children. It was dreadful artistry, but every generation of surgeons tried harder than the preceding one, using every ounce of technical and surgical wizardry, to restore a semblance of function and cosmesis to these maimed children.

The lives of these little patients had mutated from acute—where they could barely survive from one heartbeat to the next—to chronic, where their lives were less precarious. They began to endure. Like geologic formations, the children became sedimentary, surgical layers, recording each new technical era, one upheaval to the next.

To my unpracticed eye on this first day's tour, everything seemed normal for a pediatric ward. The walls were decorated with scenes where cute elephants held many-colored balloons in their trunks. Between them, clowns danced, holding hands with puppies, all skipping together down the lengths of the hallway. In the distance, I could make out children, their silhouettes whole enough. Here and there, I saw a swaying gait, suggestive of a limp. But from a distance, I never guessed something was amiss.

Up close, however, the children took my breath away. As I neared the first child, I saw that it wore a dark-tan elastic mask. I later learned these rubberized, stretchy garments were custom-fitted to each child to help smooth and flatten scar tissue. This particular mask was askew, giving the child the look of a mutant buccaneer with a single eye exposed. The globe of the child's eye was tethered to one corner of a red, angry socket. The eye itself was a deathly, milky white, plain as marble. The iris had lost all color. The left ear was completely gone, melted like a forgotten candle, leaving only a dark canal leading menacingly into the skull.

I could extrapolate where the lips had been. The nose was gone. On the left hand, there were remnants of fingers and a nubbin of a thumb. More akin to a catcher's mitt. The child's limbs were bent at odd angles, webbed across the joints with dense, contracting scars. But the voice! The voice was so clear! The essence of a child's singsong tones. I was oddly relieved that a child was indeed residing in this misshapen anatomy.

I struggled to regain my composure as the nurse led me to another bed. We proceeded with increasing speed, from one bedside to the next. Her storytelling accelerated—a vignette for each apparition.

It went on, making me heartsick, even angry that the world could be such a dangerous place for children. At the same time, I wished for a spiritual heroin, to ease my own sorrow.

It took me weeks to settle down. In the earliest part of the rotation, I was relieved just to get out of the Burn Institute, to breathe a lungful of air, free from antiseptic. I would gaze at people walking down the street, with hands as smooth and perfect as porcelain. Bodies like supple saplings. It amazed me how utterly normal the physical world was outside.

Going inside Crispy Critters each day was like being condemned, my heart drowning as soon as I passed through the doors.

Over a period of weeks, I got to know each child. I learned it was easier for the children to become assimilated into the surgical world than into the real one. With time, each child realized it was safer inside than out. At first, they were unaware of their horrific appearance. The children would believe their well-intentioned social workers, teachers, or parents who promised them they could return to normal life. These adults would try to pave the way—to soothe the furrowed and recoiling faces that lined the sidewalks, store aisles, and playgrounds of the children's earlier lives before they had been burned. But how could anyone prepare the unscarred world? How could anyone soften its reception? As physicians, supposedly hardened by years of witnessing such burns, we could not accustom ourselves to it. So how could civilians? How do you prepare a group of first-graders for the grisly transformation of a burned child? You can't!

But every burned child wanted to go back home. Such is a child's nature: to gravitate back to the company of playmates. So each would try once, twice, but never more than three times. Eventually, every single one came back to Crispy Critters. They'd come whimpering back to the safety of the den. Here, inside, everyone was burned or scarred. Here, the very notion of normality had mutated to something unrecognizable to the outside world.

My initial assessment was that this tragic world of scarred children was simply too sad for me to even understand. The children endured so many operations the medical staff lost count. Here, even the pain of endless surgical revisions became easier to bear than the pain of rejection in the outside world.

One child I recall vividly at Camp Chronic was named Henry. He had no less than eight volumes of medical records and had been nicknamed—you guessed it—Henry the Eighth. Henry the Eighth had lasted through a record 127 surgical procedures in less than three and a half years. What else could Henry (or any of the children for that matter) do? Should we simply have left them as they were? Should we deprive them of whatever small improvement reconstructive plastic surgery could provide? Was it better to live with lobster claws than without hands? With claws you could at least hold your crayon.

After a spell, I began to see things differently. Every child became a small, brave experiment in courage, endurance, and improvisation. Each was a spiritual prototype, sent out to test the winds of humanity's compassion. Each time a burned girl or boy left Crispy Critters, he or she would fly away. Eventually they all returned, telling us the world was still not ready. Gradually, Crispy Critters was no longer the bleak prison I had first seen. It became a hybrid of laboratory and chapel. Life had been rendered to molten form. Child after child was recast into an angel and then sent to test the world's pity. And we—the outside, unmarred world—repeatedly failed them.

Finally, one single angel-child made it. His name was Thomas. His story, like those of so many in the institute, had a grim beginning. When he was about ten years old, he and a friend were playing in the rolling farm country outside Lancaster, Pennsylvania. They walked across fields that were pushing up the green promise of the season's first corn. From there, they passed through the edge of the family farm. As they hiked, they came across a footpath to the crest of a large hill, upon which sat a tall high-tension line. The tower there commanded a view of the whole countryside. From on high, they'd see not only their own houses but even horizons far beyond.

What a view it must have been! For a moment, they must have felt like eagles. But Thomas slipped. He fell about a dozen feet down and came to an abrupt halt. His clothes had caught on one of the arms of the high-voltage tower. He reached up to pull himself off, and as soon as he touched the power line, thousands of volts arced into his small body, which shook convulsively. The flailing body tore loose from its snag, but not before his clothing had caught fire. He now plummeted more than one hundred feet to the ground, a flaming meteorite. His companion, frozen with fear, could do nothing but look down in horror at the motionless form of his friend. He was too terrified to move and clung to the electric tower, assuming the identical fate would befall him.

Smoke rising over the horizon alerted firefighters to the spot. More than once, kids had carelessly built a campfire that could easily spread to the adjoining woods. The firefighters arrived on the scene quickly. They rescued Thomas's friend and lowered him safely to the ground. Of Thomas, there remained little that was not burned. Only the usual small patches of intact skin remained in the axillae, groin, and the folds of certain joints. It seemed as if every bone had been broken. Nearly all the soft organs were damaged and bleeding. No one held much hope the boy could survive. Mercy dictated that dying might have been gentler.

Thomas's life, however, continued to flicker. The paramedics stabilized the boy and got him to a trauma center in Philadelphia. He underwent three operations there to stem the internal bleeding. Then the doctors were faced with the daunting task of how to get his body resurfaced with skin. That was when he arrived at the Shriners Burn Institute and became my patient.

A special medical turboprop aircraft brought Thomas to Boston. He landed ready to enter Mummy World, swaddled from head to toe in gauze. Intravenous lines poked in and out of the dressings like unruly vines. He was whisked by ambulance to a cubicle in the Shriners ICU. In the initial phases of critical burn care, the victim must be covered with new skin. This is first accomplished with grafts taken from fresh cadavers. Although the skin is dead, the thin strips of dermis and epithelium work beautifully as temporary skin. Soon the patient's immune system rejects the foreign grafts. The hope is that the cadaver grafts will buy enough time that the remaining pieces of the patient's own skin—called "autologous" skin—can be gradually harvested to resurface the body. Since these latter grafts are taken only from the patient's own cells, the body has no need to reject them.

Thomas's body had an unusually potent proclivity for rejecting cadaver grafts. While in most cases a patient might reject a graft in ten to fourteen days, Thomas would slough his off within five. We'd have to find more skin in the hospital's tissue bank. Then we'd attempt to resurface his whole body again. Each time it required six to eight hours of tedious work to suture the new skin grafts into place.

It was painstaking and wearying surgery. There was something gruesome about skinning a human corpse. It was grotesque to sew new skin into place like upholstery fabric. But there was little else we could do to save Thomas's life. The second series of grafts was rejected in just four days. We undertook a third set, and a fourth set. The latter lasted less than forty-eight hours.

Thomas wasn't likely to survive. We simply couldn't harvest enough native grafts from his armpits, scrotum, and perineum to cover his entire body surface quickly enough. It would have required months to go back and forth, lifting a graft from each small, unburned region and then suturing it into place. Then we'd have to wait three or four weeks for new epithelium to grow back into the original harvest site before we could begin the whole process over again.

We were ready to give up on Thomas—more out of exhaustion than pity perhaps. But fate intervened. Needless to say, Thomas's family was devastated by what had happened to their son. He was burned beyond recognition. Oozing. Broken. Each day he moved closer to death. The stress on his parents was unbearable. To be isolated in Philadelphia, while their son's life slipped through our hands in Boston, proved to be too much. Thomas's father, only forty-two years old, collapsed from a heart attack and died.

Thomas's mother called us to let the surgeons and nurses know her husband had passed away. There was no way to tell Thomas, because he'd been in a coma since the firefighters had found him in Pennsylvania. It seemed to me just too much tragedy for anyone to bear. But his mother calmly asked us if we would be interested in coming to Philadelphia to harvest skin grafts from her husband's body. The idea had some merit. Thomas's condition had only worsened over the last several days. He was slipping deeper into coma with each bout of graft rejection. Already, he was becoming peppered with small abscesses and sites of local infection, signs that the current cadaveric grafts would soon be shed. But skin from Thomas's father might not be rejected—if would not be autologous tissue but it would be darn close. It was worth a shot. Actually, the only one we had at that point.

So our surgical team flew down to Philadelphia with our crates of surgical instruments. As I mentioned, harvesting skin is grisly business. We use long and very sharp knives that resemble short swords. The surgeon peels the skin away, like bark off a young tree. Looking at the gray, cold body of the father, I couldn't fathom any relationship between this lifeless form and the other near-lifeless one back in Boston. But we sliced the skin as thinly as we could and packed the translucent strips in sterile plastic bags, placed inside a refrigerated cooler for the return trip.

At the Shriners, more bad news awaited us. During the night, Thomas had worsened significantly. Bacteria were growing in his bloodstream. He was slipping into a terminal, septic coma. We felt and looked like fools, stranded on the beach with our picnic cooler full of skin. It seemed a grim, futile joke.

In the coffee-break room at Crispy Critters, we debated endlessly. Should we just freeze the father's skin and keep it in the unlikely event that Thomas might survive? The senior surgical attendings then sequestered themselves in another room. Now, as an attending myself, I can imagine their conversation. There would have been discussion about the waste of valuable resources already committed to Thomas's care. Some would bemoan the wild-goose chase to Philadelphia, to save a kid who was clearly headed down the drain. But there would also have been a voice or two pleading passionately for hope. There was one last chance: Use the skin grafts from the father.

Hope prevailed. The decision was made to take Thomas to the operating room and cover him with his father's skin. At 8:30 A.M., we removed all the dead graft tissue covering Thomas. Painstakingly, over the next eight hours, we quilted his father's skin onto him. To me, the grafts looked lifeless and gray. I had little confidence. All I could think about was all the waste. Thomas's young life. His father's. Long parts of our own lifetimes.

By dinnertime, we had finished. Fresh bandages in place, Thomas's comatose body was wheeled back into its slot in Mummy World. His vital signs seemed stable enough. We knew he'd survived considerable surgery, but we had doubts about his physiologic reserves. I went into the call room and fell asleep instantly. I had been on the move for more than forty-eight hours straight.

Only seconds seemed to pass before I woke up angry and disoriented. A nurse was knocking loudly on the call room door. I looked at my watch. I'd been asleep for over two hours. The nurse was hammering, and it suddenly flashed into my mind that Thomas was probably dying. Maybe his heart had already stopped. Maybe she was calling me to help supervise CPR. I steeled myself to be able to call it off. Let him slip away. We'd done everything possible. It was time to let go.

I opened the door. The nurse was stammering. "It's Thomas... he's...he's trying...to talk!"

That simply wasn't possible. Thomas must be having problems with his ventilator. She'd misinterpreted his respiratory efforts as an attempt to talk. Hadn't he been in a coma for nearly a month?

I went right to the ICU. Not only was Thomas trying to speak, he was moving all of his limbs—something he'd never done before. He was fighting his bandages and constraints. It must have been extremely painful, as many of the fractures hadn't yet healed. But the efforts were unmistakable. He was trying to pull the endotracheal tube out of his windpipe. Of course, his hands were wrapped in dressings and tied down. There was no way he could bend his arm enough to reach it.

I slipped my hands inside the plastic-encased arm ports and reached around his throat to undo the knot. There's a small balloon at the end of the tube that helps hold it securely in place at the top of the trachea and below the larynx. I got the tie undone and deflated the balloon. I could hear Thomas trying to move air around the deflated tube. So daring more than hoping, I pulled the tube out of his mouth.

He coughed violently a couple of times. Suddenly, he spoke. His voice was perfectly clear.

"What happened to my father?" were the first words out of his mouth.

Of course, no one had said a word to Thomas about his father. How could we? He'd been unconscious the entire time! The nurses looked at me. It was my responsibility to answer. After all, I'd been the one who removed the boy's endotracheal tube.

I decided to lie. "Nothing has happened to your father, Thomas. He's just fine," I said.

Thomas looked at me in confusion. "Are you sure?" The boy was completely lucid.

"Yes. I'm sure. He's fine. He'll be glad to hear you're getting better."

Today, I deeply regret that lie. I should have told him the truth right away. But I was a young resident. I didn't know better. I thought I was being kind. Thomas knew something was wrong.

"My dad's just standing there at the end of my bed. Why doesn't he say something?" There was the hammer blow.

For a crazy instant, I blanked out what had actually happened. The father's death. The harvest of skin. Then reality returned. Thomas must be seeing someone through the plastic, a distorted silhouette that reminded him of his dad. I looked around. No one was there. Just the drapes and the lights beyond.

"Thomas," I asked, choking back tears in disbelief, "where do you see your father?"

"He's standing right there," he answered, staring at the empty foot of the bed. "Hi, Dad!" he called out, and he feebly attempted to wave.

One of the nurses choked back a sob.

"Thomas, your dad's passed away," I admitted. "He died three days ago. He had a heart attack."

I could see the shock registering within, even beneath so many layers of bandages. Then I heard him whisper something. I leaned over.

"That must be his ghost then that's waving back at me," he said softly.

I know without a shadow of a doubt that what Thomas saw at the foot of his bed was his father's actual spirit standing there, watching over him. Here was my own fragile moment of awakening. It left me tingling all over, as if sparks were dancing off my skin.

Thomas got better. He didn't reject his father's grafts. And over the next month, a researcher at the Massachusetts Institute of Technology announced a new research method to harvest epidermal cells. The patches of skin required for this experimental technique were exactly like those Thomas had still intact. Harvested cells from these patches were taken to a laboratory, induced to grow, and spread atop a layer of denatured collagen. Eventually, the cells would coalesce on the collagen sheet and it could be grafted directly onto the patient. Since the original cells were all derived from the patient (who was now the donor and later would become the host), there was no risk of immunologic rejection. Thomas was the first patient in medical history to undergo this procedure. His survival was, in effect, the culmination of a long sequence of miracles—not the least of which was the protection his father's spirit had provided.

As the months went by, Thomas was strong enough to graduate to Camp Chronic. He went through the usual series of surgical revisions. All his fingers were gone, so he got a reconstruction that gave him something akin to lobster claws. He received a new nose constructed of fat and muscle from his scalp then covered over with a graft patch of skin. More a piece of fleshy caulking than elegant reconstruction. It seemed to cover up what was, for the average onlooker, a monstrous gap, irreconcilable with our usual notion of facial symmetry and composition. He may even have surpassed Henry the Eighth in the number of procedures endured. But he was alive. Against all odds. And his shining spirit was clear and bright.

If anything, Thomas's spirit burned brighter than others'. He became indomitable. Where hundreds of kids had faltered, he would not. He was adamant to return to public school outside Philadelphia. Then the prosthetic shoes on his feet failed. Both legs became infected, and he had to have bilateral amputations below the knee. It took four more months to learn to walk again. But he did, and then he asked to return home, back to school.

It took seven more years to complete my neurosurgical training. I lost track of Thomas. Occasionally, I'd ask an intern who rotated over at Crispy Critters if Thomas had been seen. Once, one guy said he spotted him. I still remember his affirmation—he pretended to gag himself with his finger to indicate his revulsion at the mention of his name. Inwardly, I was shocked we could approve of such callous disregard. Outwardly, I smiled. To show our collective bravery, our brotherly denial of sensibility, and our solidarity in the face of vulnerability. In residency, no one gets points for being sensitive. Being cold, resolute, and impervious is what gains you admiration in the eyes of your teammates.

I didn't see Thomas again until the very last day of my final year as a resident. Tell me that was just a coincidence too! I was on the elevator. In the corner stood a horribly disfigured, diminutive person. Next to it was an attractive woman. I suddenly recognized her. It was Thomas's mother. But I never would have known the person next to her was *him*.

Thomas didn't remember me at all. His mother did. She bragged to me that he was an honor student now. And she wept, as we departed, telling me how grateful she was for what we had done for him. He waved goodbye to me with one of his misshapened hands I had probably helped build for him.

But as he waved, he smiled at me. A big smile! A real smile! The smile of someone who is genuinely happy to be alive. Then I realized that I had been given a great gift on this very last day of my surgical training. I had been brought in a great, full circle. I had seen the hell of Crispy Critters. I had learned to see beyond the burns and the deformities to the real children who lived and thrived there. I had been permitted to experience the transformational moment when the spirit of Thomas's father had come from beyond the realm of the flesh to intervene, to protect, and maybe even to guide us as we took care of his son. Now I had been permitted to grasp the miracle from beginning to end, its entire sweep across time and space. I had not grasped its full significance. Maybe I'd forgotten a lot. So the miracle came back, like a comet inevitably making its orbit back to visit me.

As I saw Thomas smile and wave, I reminded myself I had been permitted to watch the mortal threads of my life interweave with the strands of the spiritual powers in Thomas's life. The trip had lasted precisely from the beginning to the end of my entire surgical training over eight years at the MGH. That too could not be mere coincidence.

I understood, for the first time, that the filaments of my own existence were inextricably interwoven with Thomas's, his father's, his mother's, and those of a host of other individuals. An idea began to take shape: I could see thousands of orbits, mortal and spiritual, all spun from the luminous fabric of creation. This eight-year-long adventure was not just the story of a surgical residency. It was a message: We're never solitary mortal beings. Supernatural comfort is all around us—like Thomas's father's spirit—and never leaves us alone without divine strength and protection. But without the certainty of our link to the supernatural, the burden of our individual existence can make us crazy. Thomas's eight-year experience made me realize that suffering is not the point of living. It's the background, the context, against which we discover love's power over death, over illness. Suffering is what lends love its supremacy over death.

Seven

Queen of the Gypsies

mentioned residents often have to become numb to death. In some ways, it has to be that way; training works better sometimes when you're numb. Numb is good.

Some of the patients we dealt with at the MGH were Gypsies. Although the name "Gypsy" alludes to ties back to ancient Egypt (Henry VIII banned Gypsies from his kingdom under the so-called Egyptian Act of 1531), this ethnic group is thought to have originated in India. Gradually, the Gypsies made their way to Europe via Turkey and the Middle East by the end of the ninth century. By the sixteenth century, Gypsy communities were found spread throughout the European continent and Britain. With nomadic roots, Gypsy bands and groups often remained itinerant, traveling across the countryside in covered wagons carrying out trade, tinkering, or providing entertainment in exchange for goods or currency. Gypsies often found employment as seasonal agricultural workers, notably in the harvesting of hops for beer and grapes for wine.

Over the centuries, as Gypsies roamed across Europe, they were often subjected to discrimination and persecution. As recently as the nineteenth century, the British Commons Act of 1876 was aimed at banning the Gypsy wagons traveling and camping on town commons. As late as 1968, the so-called Caravan Sites Act was also designed to specifically limit these Gypsy encampments.

Myths and legends arose about the Gypsy people, most notably that many among their number possessed magical powers, permitting them to see into the future. Reading palms and tarot cards, as well as producing charms and casting spells, became the special province of the Gypsies and especially the womenfolk.

Being readily identifiable when they rolled into towns, the Gypsies were the subject of widespread fear and prejudice. In 1596, over one hundred men and women were condemned to death in England simply for being Gypsies. In order to escape persecution in the British Isles, many Gypsy families emigrated to America in the eighteenth and nineteenth centuries. One particularly large community was established in Boston during this period. So it was not uncommon, as a resident at the MGH in 1983, to take care of a member of the Gypsy families from around the New England area.

One night, an elderly woman came into the emergency room. She'd apparently suffered a major heart attack. Her organs were failing from a prolonged absence of adequate blood flow even though her heart kept beating. She was placed in the ICU, on a ventilator. Despite valiant attempts, there was little doubt she'd die. I was not privy to exactly how the senior resident informed the family, or whether they just had a better sixth sense than anyone gave them credit for, but within hours family members started gathering in somber knots inside the waiting room, down the hall from the ICU, awaiting the end.

I don't understand how families seem to know on a visceral level when loss and tragedy are about to arrive, but many times they do. Even at times when we, as physicians, are trying hard not to tell the truth. As docs, we generally don't tell outright lies. We just don't speak the truth fully, plainly. So often, families seem to know already, before we've had a chance to break the bad news. It was no different with this Gypsy woman's family.

There was an unusual detail about this elderly, dying woman. She had the improbable family nickname of Bubbles. It seemed incongruous to hear them talking about Bubbles and then see a family member leaning tenderly over the bed rail and addressing this frail, old woman in a coma. I shared her nickname with the resident team. We all chuckled. Someone wondered if maybe in an earlier time she had been a stripper or something like that. It turned out that, in fact, she was the unofficial "Queen of the Gypsies," for the whole community that lived in Boston.

Residents soon find out that every patient we get close to can cause us to feel loss. A chunk of us can get torn away with every death we witness. When you're a young physician, there just seems to be no way to reconcile so much loss. As inexperienced physicians, we lack the emotional reserves to regain our equilibrium. Later, as we mature, the sense of loss is a sign of the connection between all of us in this mortal condition. We are, in fact, not islands, but family. It takes a while to recognize that Bubbles is our sister, or our mother. She's our child. And she is a queen in the best sense of the word.

Bubbles's family made several inquiries as to whether she would make it, emerge out of her coma. Gradually, reluctantly, we started to tell the truth. In drips and drops. Suddenly, that particular night, the family gathered around her bed and broke out stumpy, squat candles. Like a well-practiced synchronized swimming team, several relatives pulled out Zippo lighters and started lighting candles in unison.

A nurse screamed out, "Fire! Fire!"

Terrified family members visiting other patients in the ICU started screaming. I remember a woman in her thirties bending low over the bed of one ICU patient to shield the person with her own body.

Someone pulled a fire alarm. Loud ringing erupted. Bubbles's family went about their business of lighting the candles. Another nurse yelled out in panic, "Oxygen! There's oxygen in the room. It's going to explode." It was pandemonium. Some panicked individuals jumped to the oxygen knobs regulating the flow from the wall outlet. Then someone else yelled out, "No! Don't turn off the oxygen knobs! Don't touch them! You'll suffocate the patients! Don't touch the wall outlets!" It seemed not to have occurred to any of Bubbles's family members that the candles could represent a substantial fire hazard.

Another person barked out, "We've got to douse those candles! We've got to get to them! Put the damn candles out! Put them out!" The whole room took up the call. "Put the candles out! Put the candles out!"

One young man slid across the floor on both knees and began pinching out the candle flames, lashing out with both hands, snapping his fingers together like castanets. Then he found himself grappling with some of the Gypsy contingent. A contest between the Zippos and the Castanet Man.

One nurse grabbed a Dixie cup, poured herself a full cup of water, and tossed the contents out into the air over Bubbles's bed. One candle hissed in protest. She had thrown her lot in with the Castanet Man.

Someone had called Security. Who had had the presence of mind to do that in the midst of this mayhem? The only useful impulse I had felt was a desire to sprint out of the building. I mean if something is going to blow, as a general rule, I don't really want to be anywhere in the vicinity. I admit it occurred to me later how wrong it was to think of saving my own hide when so many people—patients—on vents and meds, all hooked up to intravenous tubes, wouldn't have a ghost of a chance of getting out without help.

So while I had an impulse to run, I didn't bolt. Was it against the law, I wondered? Maybe there was a regulation or statute that physicians have to rescue their patients in a fire or bomb blast? Was there a law prohibiting physicians from abandoning their patients under fire? Like being a coward in the military? Maybe they could even shoot you, as a medical deserter.

As I stood there—gallantly—the MGH security guards gang-tackled every member of Bubbles's band, and had them down with their chins shoved tightly against the floor, wedging a knee between the shoulder blades, whipping out cheap plastic cable-tie handcuffs. The candles were out. Family members gradually peeled themselves off their loved ones in the ICU. Walkie-talkies crackled. An elevator door was held open. Police officers streamed in, scanning every face with practiced scrutiny. Boston firemen huffed and puffed their way into the ICU, weighed down in full gear, Scott air packs on their backs, giant fire axes in their hands, aching for action. There was none. Just splashed-out or snuffed-out candles. And a Gypsy family in restraints.

A Catholic chaplain was summoned to the scene as well. It was none other than Father Timothy Fitzgerald—renowned as both Jesuit priest and psychiatrist (which struck many as redundant). He entered the ICU and immediately pleaded for everyone to remain calm.

It was too late for that. At least we all could try—at least try—to regain our composure. Soon we all had this wide-eyed look of surprise. As if we were saying, "What the hell? We're getting so worked up! Look at us! Going to pieces over a few little candles. And, well heck, Bubbles's family probably meant no harm. It was all harmless. Innocent, right?"

Under Father Fitz's careful shepherding, we all gradually looked at one another, shaking our heads in disbelief at ourselves, and smiled. How could we have all acted that way? So panicked? The hospital security guards even helped Bubbles's family to their feet and dusted them off politely. Patted their shirts and ties back into position. Shrugged at the handcuffs apologetically. It was, it seemed after all, a big mistake. A misunderstanding. Shoot, we're sorry. Really sorry. So what were you trying to do with those candles anyway, you crazy Gypsies?

Father Fitz hastily convened a congregation in a private conference room just outside the ICU entrance. Everybody—from the docs to the janitors—called the place "the grieving room." There was no deceiving anyone about the room's purpose. This was where you usually gave 'em the bad news.

Here a family could wail, scream, pound their fists, and vent their rage. There were no windows. For all I knew, someone had had the engineering foresight to soundproof the room too. There were two shelves in the room. One shelf held religious texts of almost every description. The Bible was there. The Koran. Texts in Hebrew. Texts about Buddha. There were two copies of *Why Bad Things Happen to Good People*. From time to time, some mysterious process would quietly add a book to the collection. A donation perhaps. A mourner who left a meaningful book for the next distraught family. It was the one and only place in the hospital where books never got ripped off. Either out of a sense of sanctity or pragmatism. The grieving room was hallowed ground in the otherwise ruthless world of the MGH. Or perhaps there was simply no interest. Who'd want to read religious texts in the hospital unless someone in their family was dying?

The other shelf in the grieving room had Kleenex tissue boxes. Not one or two for backup. No, there were at least a hundred boxes. It looked as if a forklift had been used to meet the consumption driven by all that cumulative weeping and wailing. Again, it struck an odd chord. Yeah, it was great that they had the Kleenex there. As they taught us as medical students in Psychiatry rotations, "The clear and unobstructed view of the box of tissues tells the patient that you are giving them permission to cry, to give full expression to their emotions. The box of tissues is a permissive symbol to the patient's subconscious that with you they can give expression to their greatest fears and losses. The Kleenex tells them that they are safe with you." Yeah, right! Still, the stacks and stacks of Kleenex boxes looked like an industrial message: "You'll need five Kleenex per grieving widow. Ten if the family's got kids!"

So Father Fitz brought Bubbles's family into the grieving room along with me, Bubbles's primary nurse, and one or two hospital security guards. They felt that they had to be there because the family was still handcuffed and, therefore, technically in their custody. It was a tad uncomfortable at first, because it's hard to sit down with your arms pinned behind your back. So everyone who was handcuffed remained standing. With the family standing, none of the staff felt comfortable sitting either, so we all stood.

Father Fitz patiently questioned the family about the candles. After some skillful coaxing on his part, a family spokesperson explained that one of the Gypsies' beliefs was that a person's soul must have access to the heavens at the moment of death. If the individual cannot die outside, then candles are lit all around the bed so the soul is permitted to escape safely. It is carried upward with the smoke and heat from the candles, thus gaining immediate access to Heaven. If the soul is denied direct ascension to Heaven, well, then, the soul could wander. Some souls...well (at this point the family members looked at one another knowingly as if to say "we'd better not go there, folks"), some souls could get into mischief. And even worse. I wondered what. What could be worse then wandering in some unresolved state like a disgruntled, embittered ghost? What? Then I remembered some vague memory from my childhood, watching *Chiller Theater* on Saturday nights. Vampires! Didn't vampires have some sort of direct link to Gypsies and Transylvania? Wasn't that inhabited wholly or at least in part by Gypsies? And maybe when their souls roamed...No wonder, I thought, they would be willing to burn the entire hospital to the ground!

Father Fitz sighed with understanding. This really was one of those situations where it helped to have dual training as priest and psychiatrist. I looked over his garb. Did he have a cross hanging prominently anywhere? I remembered how vampires couldn't stand mirrors. Mirrors? Or garlic? Not garlic. Crucifixes? Darn, there wasn't even a little cross on his lapel or anything.

Father Fitz mulled over the problem in silence as he stroked his substantial gray beard. The problem, as he saw it, was that either Bubbles needed to have her soul set free or we were going to be stuck with some incendiary solution. His eyes roamed thoughtfully from family member to family member, as he looked at each one with his deeply set gaze.

"Would it, er, satisfy your needs...your beliefs...if we could make some arrangement? If it was cleared, if you could accompany her in her bed outside?" he asked, weighing each word.

"Do you mean that Bubbles could be lying in her bed and be outside?" asked one of the elder men, still with plenty of heft left in his great arms pinned behind him. The other Gypsies nodded their approval.

"Yes, I do mean in the open air. Would that do it?"

The elder looked around. Everyone nodded. "Yes, that would be okay," someone said authoritatively.

Father Fitz looked at the security guards. Was there any way? At first, it was impossible. Unthinkable! But Father Fitz was working for a higher authority, and soon one of the security guards said there was a freight elevator over on the east side of the hospital where the faculty offices were located. There, they could fit a hospital bed. They would have to cross over to the third floor, and then from there they could get up to the roof. It would be the roof over the office building. Not the roof of the hospital, if that mattered.

That was not an issue according to the family. Heaven was Heaven, after all. It extended everywhere. Father Fitz and his band of Gypsy freedom fighters had hatched a plan.

The plastic handcuffs came off. They wheeled Bubbles and her ventilator, along with a monster-sized monitor, through nearly a half-mile of corridors until they got her loaded onto the freight elevator, and eventually got her hoisted up onto the roof. From there, the guards and family members had to lift the whole bed up in the air to get it over a low escarpment.

There was only one reason I was present: I carried the code box. A dramatic, plastic toolbox filled with all sorts of cardiac ampoules full of goodies all guaranteed to jump-start any heart. The thing was, Father Fitz had had the family sign a "DNR"—"do-not-resuscitate"—order because it was felt that pulling Bubbles out of the ICU was putting her at increased likelihood of dying. Of course, she was dying anyway, so the DNR just put an end to any medical absurdities of pretending to flog Bubbles back to life just so she could die again. Father Fitz was as cunning as he was insightful. I couldn't figure out if it was the Jesuit in him or the shrink.

So Bubbles lay out on the roof of the hospital's office building with an incredible view of the skyline and Fenway Park and a great view of the Charles River, sparkling like a stream of diamonds from Boston to Newton. It was a beautiful night. It was hard to remember we were there to let this Gypsy queen die. The whole family queued up and then, one by one, each planted a kiss on her forehead or on a cheek. Seeing them pay homage to her, I could tell she had really been their queen.

She died. The monitor whined as she flatlined. Once and for all. It felt really odd. Standing there with the code box in my hand and letting her slip away. Like a leaf floating down to meet the river. Pulled away, off into the distance, she was gone. Father Fitz crossed himself. The security guards helped haul the bed back down to the freight elevator and took her body directly down to the basement, to the morgue. I got off on the third floor and walked back to the ICU. The head nurse had to recheck that the seal on the code box was still unbroken. She signed it in and put it back on the shelf. Ready for the next round. The next soul waiting in line.

The funny thing was all the residents already knew about that exact route we took up to the roof. When the summer sun was out, we'd strip down to just the pants of our scrub outfits and pull out lawn chairs to sun ourselves on that very spot. Sometimes we'd even sneak a six-pack or two up there and have a little roof party.

I could never bring myself to go back up there and get a tan where Bubbles had lain in state. Like or it not, she had ruined that for me. But the pathetic thing is it took me years before I could appreciate the dignity I had witnessed in that impromptu ritual Father Fitz had organized. What gives us a chance of standing up against death, of defying it, is our awareness. Ritual enhances insight, which, in turn, opens the doors to spirituality. Love offers humanity the only means to escape the gravitational pull of death.

Eight

Incidental Finding

S urgeons learn first by dogma and then from experience. After a few years, they find a balance point between a malady's natural progression and the damage inflicted by surgical intervention. Establishing that point for each patient is critical, because it tells a surgeon when an operative procedure can be honestly and ethically contemplated.

Every surgeon struggles with the guilty mathematics of experience. All of us are haunted by that handful of patients that gave their lives so each one of us could gain surgical experience. From them, we learn how to save others who come under our knife later. And there comes a time when achieving surgical mastery permits us to save lives in scenarios we never dreamt could be surmounted. The equation becomes sweeter: far more lives saved than were ever lost. Still, every surgeon wishes he or she could go back to resurrect a few that perished, to erase a few names on that personal, private, painful list.

In 1986, as I related earlier, I was involved in research studies for the U.S. Army on how the brain reacted to low levels of oxygen, especially the hypoxic extremes that occur when troops are deployed to high altitudes. Our goal was to find methods to assist soldiers to more rapidly adjust or acclimatize to high altitude. One of the biggest problems at high altitude is that the brain swells and individuals develop pounding, intractable headaches associated with listlessness, nausea, and vomiting.

The research protocol was complicated and arduous. I was responsible for obtaining MRI pictures of the brain as it struggled with lower concentrations of oxygen, in the thinner air at high altitudes. To do this, we had to expose several volunteers to the acute effects of hypobaria—lower atmospheric pressure—in a large high-altitude chamber. The largest chamber in the world is located just outside Boston, in Natick, Massachusetts, at the U.S. Army Research Institute of Environmental Medicine (USARIEM). In this facility we could simulate rapid ascents to over 16,000 feet above sea level. We could later repressurize the soldiers back to sea level. In order to prevent them from recovering too quickly from acute mountain sickness (AMS), we took the precaution of placing a face mask on each soldier, so they could all breathe a special mixture of nitrogen and low oxygen while we drove them to a nearby MRI imaging suite and acquired images of each brain. But with what could we compare these brain images? How about normal volunteers who had not been recently exposed to high altitude? So we decided to obtain normal control MRIs from any healthy individual between the ages of twenty and thirty who had remained at sea level for the last six months.

I became something of a regular at the MRI facility. I grew chummy with the technicians who sat at the terminals obtaining our brain images well into the night. One of the techs, named Valerie, was a sweet, attractive woman in her twenties. She had recently become engaged and had also been promoted to work as part of the MRI scanner staff. Valerie seemed to enjoy having me point out some of the anatomy that was visible on the MRI images. One night she asked me if she could be one of the sea-level controls. She thought it would be really neat to see a picture of her own brain.

"Besides," she added, "that way I'll have evidence to show to my fiancé that I do actually have a brain up there and that it's not just all air."

Since the U.S. Army was funding the study, there was no charge to the volunteers for the otherwise expensive images (one MRI cost about a thousand dollars at the time). We both thought it was a great perk for her, so I set up an appointment. I made arrangements for Valerie to be imaged right after I had finished with the next batch of altitude subjects. After the images were completed, the military subjects were allowed to sit and breathe in deeply the luxuriant air available at sea level. I always marveled at how the symptoms of AMS subsided in as little as a few minutes once the subjects were back down at sea level.

Valerie set the controls on the MRI scanner and then climbed on the table. I slid her into the machine and then started the scanning sequence of her head. The MRI went without a hitch. I downloaded the images and sent them over to a neuroradiologist at USARIEM to review the next morning.

When I got back to the Altitude Division offices the next day, there was a message taped to the handset of my telephone. It read: "Allan— Call me as soon as you get in. One of your subjects has an aneurysm. Carl." Carl was a great radiologist and I ran downstairs to his office. It was Valerie's scan. It showed an 8mm-wide aneurysm on the middle cerebral artery. An aneurysm is a small weak spot in the artery that balloons out like a thin bubble. If it ruptures, there's usually better than a 50 percent chance it will kill or permanently cripple the patient. On the other hand, if it's operated on before it ruptures, there is less than a 1 percent chance of dying.

I sat down with Valerie that evening at the MRI suite and showed her the images. I explained carefully to her why I thought she should seriously consider an operation. It was an aneurysm, already big enough to rupture. The bigger the aneurysm, the greater the chance of bursting. In that regard, an aneurysm is a lot like bubble gum. The bigger the bubble, the easier it will pop. The other thing about Valerie's aneurysm was that it was located on the left middle cerebral artery (or MCA), and that was linked to vital areas of speech and motor function—hardly a benign area in which to have an aneurysm rupture.

I recommended that she go to see one of my professors at the MGH. He was one of the country's foremost aneurysm surgeons: Alberto Contente. Aneurysm clipping is an entire subspecialty unto itself within the larger domain of neurosurgery. Alberto had huge experience and was one of the best aneurysm surgeons in the world. I had grown fond of Valerie. She did not seem to entirely grasp the gravity of the situation, but in some ways I felt that that might be better for her. She asked me a lot of questions about how much hair would need to be clipped off for the surgery. How quickly would it grow back? How soon could she dye her hair again? Things like that.

Alberto saw her and scheduled her for surgery in one week's time. He promised her to be extremely sparing with shaving hair for the craniotomy incision. He reassured her there would be no problem with getting coiffed in time for her wedding. Alberto knew I would be interested in the surgery itself, so he invited me to the OR to observe. I was flattered by the invitation. Later, I wished I'd never accepted the offer.

During the operation, Alberto was getting ready to set the little metallic clip around the neck of the aneurysm bubble. As he nestled the clip into position, the aneurysm ruptured. Exploded is more accurate. No one is more coolheaded than Alberto under such circumstances. He tried to reposition the clip again as blood overwhelmed the dissection cavity. To no avail. He plunged a larger sucker into the operative field and managed to get a temporary clip on the parent vessel. When the blood was cleared out with irrigation, Alberto could see the aneurysm had torn away from the vessel. Part of its wall was gone, and a big hole left in its place. I could see each detail on the television monitor overhead.

Alberto sighed. I felt sick. I reminded myself that no one in the world was better than Alberto. But this was going to be a daunting task. He would have to harvest a vein to serve as a patch to graft the side of the vessel back together. I also knew that such a repair carried an enormous risk to Valerie. With the rupture of the dome and neck of the aneurysm, Valerie's chance of dying had suddenly increased by fiftyfold!

It was agony to watch Alberto. He deftly, expertly carried out the repair. None of his skill changed anything. Valerie's brain began to turn a dusky, dark color. Her brain was evolving a stroke, an infarct, in front of our eyes. Alberto drove himself as fast as he could. The clip came off in under twenty minutes. That was about a world record for the fastest time ever for a vein patch. But Valerie's brain stroked. We looked on helplessly as a large amount of cerebral cortex started to die. Later, in a second, desperate attempt to save her life, Alberto brought her back down to the OR. He removed the area of stroke—now dead tissue—in the temporal lobe to help relieve the excessive pressure and swelling developing in her skull. He brought Valerie back again, a third and final time, the next morning. Eventually, we all gathered with the family and made the decision there would be no further heroic attempts. We'd lost Valerie.

Alberto and I walked to his office after the last surgery. He was devastated. I was in shock.

"You must not," he said, "blame yourself, Allan. You made the right decision to send her here. It was the right call. What happened was just fate. That's all."

"I know, Alberto. But I can't help wondering whether, if I had not consented to letting her be a sea-level subject and getting the MRI scan, no one would have known. Whether she would never have known."

"But then it would have ruptured one day."

"Who knows? Maybe. Maybe not. She might have died at the ripe old age of ninety and taken the damn aneurysm to her grave," I said.

"Or maybe she would have ruptured during childbirth, while she was in labor. There are plenty of cases in the neurosurgical literature, as you know, where women can die like that. Or maybe it would have ruptured while she was driving a bus full of children to school."

"She was an MRI tech, for Christ's sake."

"I know that. I'm just making a point," said Alberto.

"Well, tell me then: What is the point? Dying like this. Leaving a fiancé. A family. All of them bereaved over what? Over a shadow on an MRI scan."

"She died because that was just... well, it just happened the way that it happened. We both saw it."

In many ways, it is irrational for a surgeon to dedicate his life to trying to save people knowing, at the same time, that he's an instrument for dying too. Still, after Valerie's death, I took precautions. I'm superstitious, as I said earlier. So I made myself a rule: Never let anyone but a total stranger ever volunteer to be a subject for any research study of mine. I figured that the rule would ensure I would never again make a gruesome, incidental discovery in any friend of mine. It's a silly rule and hopelessly futile, of course. But it makes the world feel safer to me.

Nine

Mother-and-Child Reunion

O fairer daughter of a fair mother!

HORACE

andy was one of my close friends. And, yes, with a name like Candy, she looked like one of those gorgeous, fetching, doe-eyed blondes you used to see in *Playboy* magazine. She was a beauty. But she was also the most competent, intelligent, and compassionate nurse I'd ever met. I'd known her back in Boston, where she'd been an ICU nurse with me on Gray 11—the neurosurgical ICU at the MGH.

As beautiful and wonderful as Candy was, her life was anything but pretty. This was long before society's awareness of domestic violence had risen to the level it is at today (still grossly inadequate). I remember Candy occasionally came into work with a lot of makeup, trying to cover up a black eye or bruises on her face. As a resident I was totally clueless as to what was going on. I just accepted her excuses about falling in the basement or hitting her head on a kitchen cabinet.

By 1992, she had finally had enough of being battered and beaten by her husband and divorced him. She called me to find out about my position as assistant professor of neurosurgery at the university in Tucson. Eventually I convinced Candy to apply for a job at the Arizona Cancer Center. I was, needless to say, ecstatic to recommend her to the director of Nursing.

So Candy left her abusive past behind and moved to Tucson and began a new life. She bought herself a modest house. Her oldest boy, Sean, was already a freshman at Boston College, so he had remained behind to finish out the year. Taylor, her fifteen-year-old daughter, came with her and enrolled in the Rincon Foothills High School. Taylor was as attractive as her mom and became popular overnight—a cheerleader and the fancy of many a high school boy, I'm sure.

In her new role as an oncology nurse, Candy also became an instant favorite around the whole institution. Patients loved her. Families of the patients loved her. And the doctors loved her. And there wasn't a single eligible bachelor in the medical center who hadn't heard about her.

Because Candy was the nurse coordinator for the Cancer Center, with dozens of patients with brain tumors, our paths crossed regularly. In fact, Candy organized the first patient-based brain tumor support group in Tucson. That was typical of her. She always found ways to gather more resources for the patients and their families. She was the epitome of the nurse who constantly advocates for her patients' needs.

It was an almost daily occurrence for us to review mutual patients and ensure everything was flowing smoothly between surgery and oncology. I respected her judgment immensely. And she finally shared with me why she had left her husband and Boston.

Sean was doing well in college, and Taylor had been recently elected homecoming queen at her new high school. After about a year in Tucson, Candy met a special, new man: Tim. He was a construction worker, and Candy gradually, cautiously, let the relationship blossom. Over the course of several months, she talked more about her growing relationship with Tim. I met him occasionally in the cafeteria when they got together for lunch. Soon there was an engagement ring on her finger. She was a happy blushing bride again.

Tim was exactly what Candy needed. He was utterly devoted to her. I shudder to think what he'd have done to anyone who dared hurt her. Candy's life seemed to be coming together. Taylor adored her new stepfather. Because Sean was a very gifted basketball player at Boston College, we had no trouble making arrangements with Carl Weston, the Arizona

Wildcats' assistant coach, to have him transfer with a full basketball scholarship to the University of Arizona. Tim built a small guesthouse adjacent to their home so Sean would have his own quarters. Then tragedy struck.

Initially, nobody knew the ambulance call into our Emergency Department in Tucson involved Sean. It was just another traffic injury. There are dozens a year along the windy stretches of Route I-10. Young kid. Massive head injury. Just outside Sierra Vista. About sixty miles south of Tucson. Sean's car was hit by a trailer that had come loose from the truck that was towing it. Heartsick, Candy called me at two in the morning. I rushed to meet her at our hospital.

The news was not good. Sean had suffered multiple contusions (bruises) of his brain. There was a large blood clot along the left hemisphere that required immediate surgery. Over the course of four hours, the neurosurgery team removed the clot and repaired a torn vein in the Sylvian fissure. The prognosis remained grim. Candy never left his side in the hospital for days. But eventually it was clear that Sean would pull through.

Like many victims of severe head trauma, he'd never be the same, however. For a while there was even some doubt about whether he would make a meaningful recovery. His right side was substantially weaker than his left, and his speech was badly disrupted. He had to go through a long rehab. But Candy and Tim had such faith in God and in Sean, they refused to give up. Coach Weston reassured them that when Sean was ready, the scholarship to attend the University of Arizona was still his—whether he could ever play again or not. Weston is a classy coach and human being.

Sean made slow, steady progress. But he was not the same Sean. Because of his frontal injury, he'd fall into angry fits of temper quicker than a rattlesnake. A minor problem in a small child. Downright dangerous for the caregivers of a powerful, athletic nineteen-year-old. Eventually, Tim modified the guesthouse so Sean could come home to live with them at last. It was not easy attending to all the problems of his recovery, but Candy took it in stride. She told me she considered her burden a blessing because it put her more in touch with her cancer patients and the struggles of their families. That was Candy to a T!

About a year rolled by with nothing much to report except the time when a bully called Sean a "retard." Sean punched the fellow hard in the face, shattering his jaw. Candy and I had to go to court to get him excused from an assault-and-battery charge. That was a close one, but the judge was very understanding and sympathetic to Sean's plight.

Fate was ready to deliver its next hammer blow. Less than a year later, Taylor was brought into the ER following an auto accident. At first, there were all the usual suspicions. Teenage female behind the wheel. It must be alcohol or drugs. But the toxicology and drug screens all came back negative. Nothing there.

Taylor insisted the accident had happened because she'd lost control of her foot on the brake. She said the entire left side of her body had gone numb. C. Miller Fisher, one of the world's greatest neurologists, used to preach to us residents back in Boston, "The truth is always at the patient's bedside." And so it was for Taylor.

She was admitted to Neurology for evaluation of a stroke. I thought to myself: A ministroke? In an eighteen-year-old? Does that ever happen? I saw her in her hospital bed on the sixth floor. Her neurological exam was perfect. Absolutely no deficit. Still, I was concerned about the numbness. Seemed to me like a textbook case of thalamic stroke. But Taylor was way too young for strokes.

The thalamus is a significant sensory relay station located near the center of each hemisphere. Sensory events in the thalamus tend to present themselves as hemisensory phenomena, meaning they occur on one half, or side, of the body. Taylor reported how she had felt the numbness creep up to her face just before the accident. There was little doubt that whatever had happened to Taylor, it had taken place in her thalamus on the right side of her brain. She had described tingling over the entire left side. The brain is "crossed" with the right hemisphere governing the left side of the body. Her description was unfailingly accurate.

Certain benefits come with being a faculty member of the Department of Surgery. A junior radiology resident did the MRI scan for me stat. On the spot! But the results were ominous. A huge mass, probably a tumor, appeared to have lodged itself in Taylor's right thalamus—not a structure where anyone can safely operate. We can get a biopsy there with a thin, needlelike probe, using a sophisticated computer-guidance system (borrowed from the defense industry). But even that procedure is hazardous. Still, we needed to find out what the mass was, get a diagnosis, and start treating it. As the surgical saying goes, "When tumor is the rumor, then tissue is the issue."

I was expert at using computer-guidance systems for neurosurgery, so I was not surprised that Candy asked me to do the biopsy procedure. And I would put my stereotactic team up against any other anywhere in the world. They were second to none. So I asked my team to meet with me in my office.

We studied the MRI images. Larry Hollis, who manages our computer systems and the imaging database, asked lots of questions about which trajectory would be the safest, which one would permit us to land in a relatively silent part of the thalamus and still get a good core sample of tumor.

There would be little margin for error. We would need to enter the brain in a relatively posterior location and then skirt past the motor cortex, where all the muscle coordination for the body lies. Then we'd have to slip seamlessly through millions of motor cell cables and sensory cells to gain access to a structure called the pulvinar. This was where the tumor seemed to have its epicenter. We plotted four different trajectories and Larry looked them over on the computer. All four lay within one millimeter of one another! In other words, no matter how we traced it, our trajectory through Taylor's brain could not vary by more than the thickness of a pencil lead.

The team had done hundreds of biopsies together, but this was definitely going to be one of the more challenging cases. There was little doubt we would get the job done, but could we get it done right?

I explained to Candy and Taylor what we had come up with to reach this deep lesion, lying in a virtually impenetrable part of the brain. Taylor cried mostly. All the talk about approaches, cortex, axonal fibers, white matter tracts...it was overwhelming. Like Valerie back in Natick, she asked how much of her head would be shaved. Like her mom, she had long, golden-blond hair.

One of the advantages of computer guidance is that you know within a millimeter exactly where you need to drill through the skull. In fact, the incision for this kind of surgery is less than half the width of the nail on your pinky finger. We close it up with a single stitch and cover it with one of those dot Band-Aids, so I could reassure Taylor she wouldn't lose any hair. No one would even be able to see the incision unless she pointed it out. That brought a big smile to her face. But I knew how much of a struggle it was for Candy to see her daughter's life turned over to my team's hands—no matter how competent we might be.

The day for surgery arrived. This kind of biopsy is dangerous, so it's actually safer to perform it under local anesthesia. Taylor would feel no discomfort, but could report if she felt anything as we passed the probe into position. Her head was held rigidly in place in a metal frame. Naturally, though, being wide awake meant she would be anxious, vulnerable to the chilling atmosphere of the operating room. It's a lot to ask of anyone, especially a teenager.

Taylor was an angel. We inserted the probe cautiously, millimeter by millimeter. She told us if she felt anything. In fact, she reported only a small tingling while I was taking the tissue sample from the pulvinar. That was reassuring, because it told me the probe was correctly placed. We got our biopsy and "got out of Dodge," as we say in the business.

One of the great secrets of surgery, which no mentor can teach, is knowing when to stop a surgical procedure, to call an end to it. It's such a tough call—when to keep pushing onward and when you've gone too far. So often, a surgical outcome depends on where to call a halt. When to let the patient recover from the intrusion. Because surgery is just that—an intrusion on the body. Getting great results from surgery is less about retreat than it is about declaring a truce between the surgeon's assault and the body's defenses. Getting out at the right moment is half of a successful surgical outcome.

A postoperative scan confirmed that we had been "BDO" ("balls dead on"—an expression that came from Larry's artillery background before he came to computer navigation in surgery). There was a tiny bubble of air where the biopsy had come from. It would disappear in a matter of hours. But it showed us exactly where our specimen had been taken. We'd been right in the heart of the tumor. And Taylor was ecstatic about her tiny incision.

The news from neuropathology, however, was not good. The tumor was an anaplastic astrocytoma—a high-grade malignant brain cancer. And inoperable. We'd have to depend on radiation and chemotherapy. Candy marshaled all the resources of the Cancer Center. Anyone with any expertise in the treatment of these tumors was called on to help with Taylor's therapeutic regimen.

Taylor's beautiful golden locks inevitably fell out with the treatment. This exquisite young woman became bald, bloated, and acne-ridden. An unhappy caricature of herself wrought from steroids and chemo-therapy. At a time when most young adults are tortured enough about self-image, Taylor was transformed in front of my eyes. It was like being in a horrible fairy tale where a spell is cast upon the beautiful princess.

It's difficult even today to recall those dark days when Taylor would return for a clinic visit. A photograph of her had been taken at the begin-ning of treatment for identification purposes. It was in the front of her chart. I would always look at it before stepping into the exam room, just to remind myself how she had looked before, how I wanted to see her. I needed to remember the real Taylor that was now hidden. Worse news: the tumor did not respond. Soon her entire left side was badly affected. She could no longer feel where she was placing her feet. This gifted, acrobatic cheerleader now could barely shuffle down the hallway with a walker. As her left side got weaker, even her smile became crooked and began to look like a sneer.

Taylor never lost her sweetness, though. I will never forget one afternoon when she sat next to Candy as we all looked at yet one more MRI. It showed clearly that the tumor was growing ever larger despite all our great therapies and best intentions. She looked over at her mom.

"It's too bad I didn't know about this tumor earlier. I wouldn't have been so reluctant to give up my virginity. Now I'm probably going to die a virgin, looking the way I do."

She said it without bitterness, but it broke our hearts. It reminded us of the full impact of all the things Taylor would miss: the joy and passion of being beautiful, enjoying her body's urges, going off to college, getting married, having a career, children. With all her pent-up mother's rage, Candy muttered aloud, "Don't worry. You're not missing much. Losing your virginity is not all it's cracked up to be anyway."

Taylor died less than two months later. Janey and I attended the funeral. There was a huge crowd. Sean was there with his arm wrapped around his mother, and Tim, his weeping eyes behind sunglasses, squeezed Candy's hand throughout the ceremony. Over two hundred folks showed up from Tim and Candy's church, where they had been holding weekly prayer groups on Taylor's behalf. No sweeter child has been ripped from the bosom of a family and community. I wept for Candy and every parent who lost a child under my care.

Even after Taylor's death, however, the ordeal still wasn't over. Only a few months later, I received a hushed phone call from Candy. She was whispering, as if someone might overhear us.

"Allan, I know this sounds crazy, but I was just in the shower and I could feel the hot water on one side of my body—my left side—but I couldn't feel it on my right. I didn't know what else to do but call you." She sounded desperate.

"Listen, Candy, it's probably nothing. It may be a psychological reaction to losing Taylor. But just so we'll both feel better, I'll make arrangements for an MRI. That way you'll relax a little, and then we can deal with this."

We set it up for the next day. There are no words to explain how I felt when I went downstairs and saw an MRI scan virtually identical to

Taylor's. First, of course, I accused the radiology techs of getting the X-ray folders mixed up, but I could see Candy's name printed on one set of film plates and Taylor's on another. Besides, the date printed on each sheet of Candy's images was clearly three months after Taylor had passed away.

So there it was, staring me in the face. Candy had a brain tumor in exactly the same place as her daughter. I spent the next few hours scouring the Internet and the library for any other similar cases in medical literature. I had my staff wake up the head of the National Familial Brain Tumor Registry in Baltimore, to ask him if he had ever seen or heard of a case like this. If anyone should know, he should. He had been collecting cases of familial brain tumors all his life.

"Yeah, we've seen somewhat similar cases. But not like this—you know, not exactly in the same place. One was two brothers. Both came down with the same brain tumors within three or four years of each other. Also a father and an uncle. So it certainly can run in families."

I called Tim to have him meet me at my office rather than in the clinic. And I paged Candy to come over. She must have thought it was to talk about a mutual patient care issue. But as soon as she walked in and saw us, she clasped her hands to her mouth and started moaning, "Oh, no, no, no!" She seemed to curl up in a ball. Tim ran to her side and wrapped his body around hers, as if to shield her. I didn't have to say a single word. She knew. Later, she told me that instantly, when she had felt the shower's warmth on only one half of her body, she already suspected the terrible truth.

We went down the same path we had gone down with Taylor. First, there was the biopsy. Same results. Radiation and chemo. The same ugly transformation of a beautiful woman. Yet it never occurred to Candy to rail against her fate. She spent all her time preparing Tim to be alone, making sure Sean and Tim would be there for each other. I remember once, when we were going over some issues about chemotherapy and scans, she paused to say how glad she was she had found Tim, the true love of her life.

"I only regret that our falling in love has brought him so much pain and loss."

I told her I was sure Tim wouldn't trade a minute of it. I knew how he felt about Candy.

There's not much more to tell except to say that Candy, Tim, and I called one another almost every day just to check in. Candy lived for two and half years more. She was an inspiration to every doctor, nurse, and patient who crossed her path. She continued teaching Sunday school, about the universal love and kindness that God showers on us all, up until a week before she died—when she was finally too ill for Tim to carry her into church anymore.

We buried Candy next to Taylor. As I write this, and relive the events, they again seem almost unbearable to me. I had asked Candy once how, with so much visited upon her, she had managed. She simply answered, "The Lord never gives us more burden than we can bear." But I have to admit that, at times, it has been more than I personally could bear, watching it happen to someone close. I've been lost in tears and anger, knowing I had no right when Candy and Tim were so strong. There were moments when I felt embittered toward God for what had happened to Taylor and Candy.

Candy made me feel quite ashamed of myself every time I let my anger rise to the surface. If I asked her how God could let this happen, she would look at me very sternly.

She'd cock a finger at me, shake it, and say, "Don't you dare blame God for this! Maybe this had to happen so you'd be more motivated to help find a cure! Or maybe this was meant to test my love for Tim and Tim's love for me. But God's not to blame here!" She was furious that I ever doubted God's love for her or for me.

Tim and I stayed friends for years. He never was interested in another woman. He told me Candy was the perfect woman. He just thanked his lucky stars that a beautiful woman like her had loved him. And once, over a few too many beers, he admitted two things to me. First, there hadn't been a single day since he buried Candy that he didn't wake up and weep till he was almost too weak to stand.

The second confession was that he had wanted to kill himself at first. And would have, but for his solemn promise to Candy to look after Sean. He said keeping that promise was hard, because every day he stayed alive was one more day that he was apart from her.

"If I ever abandoned Sean, Candy would be madder and meaner than a junkyard dog, and you know Candy," he added. "When she got mad she could stay mad for a real long time. Maybe for all of Eternity. And I just couldn't stand her being mad at me. I want her to be happy to see me, when I get there. I want her to smother me with kisses and fall into my arms. So I guess I love her enough to keep on living even when I don't want to."

In more than two decades of brain tumor surgery, I have never heard of two cases quite like Candy's and Taylor's. To me, they are just one single, dreadful case.

As of 2006, however, the data from the National Familial Brain Tumor Registry now contains more than two hundred familial cases. Many occur between blood relatives, but some have also happened between a parent and a stepchild, or between stepsisters in the same household. Many of these cases cannot be traced to genetics. They probably arise from living in the same house and being exposed to the same environmental influences.

Environmental influences, such as living near the tremendous electromagnetic fields generated by high-voltage power lines, seem to be implicated. One recent study showed that electrical power-line workers in Scandinavia have more brain tumors than the average population. Another study has shown that exposure to petrochemicals could also be a risk factor. There was a study that looked at which professions had the highest incidence of brain tumors. The worst profession was that of a dentist, because they're constantly getting exposed to X-rays as they shoot film for dental radiographs. The safest profession? Bartender. Go figure.

There is some foreboding data suggesting that the electromagnetic fields generated by cellphones may be setting the stage for a whole new generation of malignant brain tumors in the decades ahead. What do we do? I don't know. I'm a cellphone junkie. So are my wife and all my kids.

A year after Candy's death, a man from Globe, Arizona, brought his wife to see me, as she had been recently diagnosed with a malignant brain tumor. Less than three months later the husband was also diagnosed with the same kind of tumor. They had worked together most of their adult lives, running a dry-cleaning business. Together with the Familial Brain Tumor Registry, I pored over the invoices from the business and found that both husband and wife had been exposed to well over a dozen potent, cancer-causing chemicals in their cleaning business.

"Why hasn't anyone said anything about these chemicals? Look at what it has done to us!" the husband cried.

In large part because of these unusual familial groupings, the U.S. government has finally undertaken a serious epidemiologic evaluation of environmental and chemical toxins and their role in the induction of malignant brain tumors. In 2004, the world's largest biomolecular consortium, under the leadership of several world-class researchers such as Jeff Trent and Mike Behrens, has begun to unravel the mystery of what genes in our own brain's cells might be triggered to start malignant astrocytomas growing. When some progress has been made in this research, we may finally have the tools we need to understand how such a disease can be visited upon families, on households.

I try, as Candy exhorted me, not to blame God. I try to understand that the Creator is helping us feel our way toward a genetic understanding of this disease. I pray that God will guide the greatest minds in research and the strongest captains of bioindustry to unlock these secrets. But I also know that God intended for the human race to be careful with Mother Earth. I know that God expects us to be more attentive stewards of our planet—His creation. Pollution is a sin frequently paid for with the blood of innocents like Candy and Taylor. And maybe yours and mine too.

Ten

The Exorcist

The graveyard is full of people who thought they were indispensable.

CHARLES DE GAULLE

I n 1991 when I was just getting started again after Desert Storm as an attending neurosurgeon in Arizona, Alfred Church came into my care. He was thirteen and had just finished a wonderful summer at camp. His family was not rich. His mama cleaned houses, and his father, endowed with a mellifluous tenor voice, made radio commercials. Alfred had a sister named Alexandra, and they all lived in a large trailer in the community of Largo, thirty miles outside Tucson.

Alfred's dad got the chance to create a radio ad campaign for a Christian camp in the mountains of northern Arizona near Prescott. Evergreen forests spread out from there for hundreds of miles along the western plateau, interrupted only by the gash of the Grand Canyon. He was so taken with the activities and recreation offered in the advertisement he had done for Camp Piney Woods that he worked extra jobs as a deejay to earn enough money to send his son the next summer.

Alfred took to life in the woods. He rode horses. Hiked. Built campfires. Learned to shoot a gun. And a bow. He grew tall, bronzed, and sinewed. He became a fine archer—one of the best the camp had ever seen. As his arms and shoulders grew in strength, he progressed to heavier, more demanding bows. Before the end of the camp season, he was shooting so well the archery counselor let him practice with a custom-made fifty-pound pull bow.

The highest award a junior bowman at camp can achieve is called the American Archer. It can only be won by scoring over two hundred points in under five rounds of six arrows with the targets standing at a distance of fifty yards away. There are few greater achievements in archery. Even some Olympic gold medalist archers have failed to qualify for the American Archer Award.

As Alfred practiced, the camp buzzed with excitement. No camper had ever tried for the American Archer. Even the archery counselor himself couldn't win it. But Alfred might. On the day he hiked up to the archery range, a fifty-yard distance had been carefully marked off. If he was successful, it would qualify officially for the American Archer Award. Brand new target covers had been put up so each arrow's placement could be unequivocally assessed for the record. The counselor had personally inspected the arrows to make sure the shafts were straight and true. He tested the feathering to make sure it was secure. An official archery referee was present to officiate. Everything was ready for the anticipated record performance.

Alfred strode up and strung the huge fifty-pound recurve bow. And the worst possible thing happened: he started to miss. Badly. His score was far too low to be even considered. He was faced with trying again— next year. Alfred was devastated. He fumed, insisting there was a reason why he'd shot so poorly. It wasn't his fault! Something had gone wrong with his right arm that day. Of course, everyone assumed he was just trying to explain away a bitter disappointment.

Alfred's failure would have just faded into the overall background of his almost-perfect summer had it not been for one attentive pediatrician. Something in the tone of Alfred's voice, the seriousness of his outrage, made the physician wonder if there hadn't been a malfunctioning of his right arm. The pediatrician wanted to look deeper, to make sure.

Upon closer physical examination, the doctor found Alfred was right: there was a small but demonstrable difference in strength between muscles on the left and the right, the right side being weaker. It was all the more noticeable because Alfred was right-handed and should have been slightly stronger in his dominant arm. Especially after a whole summer of training intensely for archery. And there was another disturbing anomaly: Alfred's reflexes in his right arm and right leg were noticeably increased over the left—a sign of something going wrong in the brain. There was no reason the reflexes should not be symmetrical.

The boy was telling the truth: his right arm wasn't functioning properly. A CT scan and an MRI were taken. There was a large tumor in the boy's brain stem. So Alfred was sent to see me. Nothing had been communicated to his family other than that Alfred might need more definitive testing. Reevaluating the neurological examination, I noticed there were also problems with the nerves exiting out of the brain stem. I reviewed the MRI scans. An ominous mass was distorting the brain stem from within. There was no doubt it was a glioma, and it was probably a malignant one.

As I reviewed the images with Alfred and his parents, I could see disbelief creeping into their faces. Alfred seemed the picture of health. How could such a monster be lurking in the most essential part of his brain? His only symptom was a miss when trying for an archery award! They needed time to digest everything. I sent them home and told them to come back in the next day or two for follow-up. Forty-eight hours later, they were back. Surprise and denial had been replaced by sorrow. Alfred, however, seemed oblivious.

The most pressing business was to obtain a histological diagnosis, and this required a biopsy. At that time in medicine, few oncologists would treat a brain stem tumor without a tissue diagnosis confirming the presence of a tumor. Nowadays, with increasingly sophisticated MRI scans, the need for biopsies in the brain stem has become less important. And that's good: there are few procedures in neurosurgery more daunting than getting a biopsy of the brain stem—because it's so full of important neurological functions. We call it "tiger country." There's hardly a surgical move that doesn't hurt the patient. Even a piece of tissue no larger than the tip of a ballpoint pen contains some vital function. There's no such thing as a safe brain stem biopsy—just a less dangerous one. We generally say a surgeon doesn't "perform" a brain stem biopsy as much as "get away" with one.

The patient is affixed to a precisely machined head ring made of titanium. It's attached, under local anesthesia, by four pins directly to the bone of the skull. It must be absolutely unmovable. The patient then undergoes CT and MR imaging with the head ring in place. A sophisticated software program allows the surgeon to pick out the target. These coordinates get transferred back precisely onto the ring. A tiny hole is drilled into the skull at the exact entry point picked out by the computer program. A foot-long probe is slid into position. It passes down through the substance of the brain stem, almost to the hilt. The patient is awake so that brain stem function can be assessed intraoperatively (as we had also done in Taylor's and Candy's cases for the thalamic biopsies).

Each time the probe moved into position, Alfred's speech would become noticeably slurred. That told me that I was passing right through the area that governed the musculature of his tongue. I pushed deeper. From the computer coordinates I knew I should be close to the center of the tumor's mass. I carefully took a small piece. When I withdrew the biopsy cannula, Alfred's speech immediately cleared, returning to normal. I placed a second probe to get a confirmatory piece. His speech slurred again, but we obtained a second piece. The frozen pathology came back compatible with a high-grade malignant glioma. We'd found what we needed to know.

Since I already had the diagnosis in a matter of minutes, I rushed to confer with the radiation oncologists. I wanted to employ the head ring already on Alfred to deliver a deep, sharply focused beam of radiation into the heart of the tumor, a computer-guided technique called stereotactic radiosurgery. It took some doing, but because the tumor was unresectable, everyone understood the potential benefit of an additional boost of radiation.

Alfred was a little groggy when we finally removed the head ring, but we were all happy to have achieved both diagnosis and treatment in less than eight hours. I decided to wait till morning to regroup with the family and consultants from the different specialties.

Both parents were in shock. His mother cried continuously, and the strain on his father's face was telling. I was also deeply affected. Alfred was the same age as my own son. How would I feel if someone suddenly announced that my child's entire future was simply not ever going to happen? Alfred's life expectancy had dropped from eighty-five years of age to fourteen overnight. In all likelihood, he wouldn't live to graduate from high school.

Alfred underwent the usual six-week course of radiation treatments. As always, this was followed by a long course of chemotherapy and steroids. His hair fell out. His weight, under the incessant appetite stimulus of steroids, ballooned up to nearly two hundred pounds. He also broke out in a raging case of acne from the steroids. Another brain tumor–induced disfiguration before my eyes.

The tumor resisted everything we threw at it. Alfred lost control of his legs and became confined to a wheelchair, although he could still stand with assistance. His high school decided that it was becoming too uncomfortable for the other children to sit in class with him. Besides, they told me, they had decided that in his present condition, Alfred represented "too much of a liability for us to oversee in a standard school environment."

I asked the school principal why he was afraid to have Alfred in school.

"He could have a seizure. He could fall out of his wheelchair, hit his head and..."

"And?"

"Well, that would be devastating."

"Even if he had a seizure or hit his head, what's the worst that could happen?" I asked.

"He could end up in the hospital.... He could..."

"Alfred's already in the hospital nearly half the time. You're worried he's going to die, right?"

"Well, yes, of course. If he were to die while at school, we would all feel terrible," the principal said.

"But he's already dying. The only thing that he cares about is going to school."

"I'm sorry, but it's out of the question. We're more than ready to set up home tutoring for Alfred. But he cannot come back to school."

"What if I write a letter to the School Board, completely indemnifying them? Could he come back on that basis?"

"No. I'm afraid our decision is final."

So amid all his suffering and indignities, Alfred was banned from school. In retrospect, I may have been too quick to protest in the face of the board's ignorance and fear. My anger did nothing except perhaps reinforce their resolve to stand by their position. Alfred's spirits never rebounded from that social shun. When his social life—in the form of his schoolmates and learning—was stripped from him, so was every reason to live.

His good will began to erode. He became more sedentary. He stayed home, eating as much as his steroid-fueled appetite would permit. As his depression became more profound, the tumor progressed. His steroid dose was raised. As the steroids climbed, his appetite grew. He could eat prodigiously. Three or four cartons of ice cream at a sitting. Soon, he hardly cared whether his school tutor came by or not. Anyway, he figured out he wasn't going to live long enough to need any education. He sat on the couch and watched game shows.

If ever there was a plague visited upon a family, Alfred's tumor was it. His sister felt as though her own schoolwork and her life had been totally eclipsed in the eyes of her parents by her brother's malady. She began looking for the attention she longed for with teenage boys from the high school. And Alfred's parents' marriage was shattering under the strain.

Alfred's mother sank into a deep depression. She began to correspond in several Internet chat rooms about alternative cancer therapies. Some individuals offered solace. Some advice. Many were scientifically rigorous and legitimate. Others advertised outlandish cure rates and preposterous hypotheses to boost their sales. One of the gals at the beauty parlor had mentioned to Alfred's mom that a relative had added shark cartilage to her diet because it had been proven to stop cancerous tumor growth. And there was a small—tiny—kernel of truth to the statement.

In the early 1970s, Judah Folkman's lab had been searching for compounds that might halt tumor progression by preventing angiogenesis, as I explained in an earlier chapter. One such material that seemed to inhibit tumor invasion was intact cartilage. It is one of the few tissues in the human body that lives directly off nutrients in the neighboring joint fluid and steadfastly prevents blood vessel ingrowth so it can remain blood-free when serving as a frictionless weight-bearing surface in articulated joints. So it came as no surprise to Folkman's team that cartilage (and shark's skeletons are an abundant source for scientific study, as their large skeletons are made entirely from cartilage) could prevent tumors from invading it. So the word spread quickly— but inaccurately—that eating shark cartilage could stop cancer. The problem with ingesting shark cartilage is that one also has to digest the cartilage. Then stomach acid completely breaks it down, just as it does when you eat a bit of the joint cartilage while chewing on your drumstick from KFC. Broken down into its constituents in the digestive tract, shark cartilage is just a smelly way to add protein to your diet. It no longer has any properties to inhibit tumor progression.

Nonetheless, businesses sprang up overnight for processing and selling huge quantities of powdered shark cartilage as a dietary supplement to cancer victims. Millions of dollars' worth of shark cartilage were being sold unregulated over the counter, and manufacturers' guidelines called for ingesting literally pounds of the gritty, malodorous powder at more than 1,000 percent markup. The profits were enormous. The demand desperate. And the suppliers unscrupulous. Alfred's mother threw herself into a frenzy of Internet searches, convincing herself that shark cartilage offered her son his only chance to be cured. Eventually, she mortgaged her family into irretrievable debt to pay for the pounds of shark cartilage she ordered for her son's consumption. All to no avail.

As an aside, I want to make it clear that I am a proponent of so-called alternative medicine. I wholeheartedly support my friend Andy Weil's program in Integrative Medicine at the University of Arizona. I've also led a half-dozen research trials to evaluate promising alternative therapies. When a patient or family needs help or advice on how to navigate their way through the labyrinth of hype and hope that is alternative medicine today, I am sympathetic and supportive.

Much of today's traditional medicine started off as the alternative therapy of yesteryear. Whenever a physician or surgeon scoffs (which many—too many—still do) at alternative medicine, I remind them of the heroic, tragic story of Ignaz Philipp Semmelweis, known in medical history as the "savior of mothers." It is a sad tale of how traditional medicine can turn its back on alternative therapies, even when they clearly are shown to be superior to established practices.

In the mid-nineteenth century, Semmelweis, a Hungarian, was relegated to delivering obstetrical care in the charity wards and poorhouses of Vienna. Hundreds of thousands of women died from infection there each year, of so-called puerperal fever, an infection occurring after childbirth. There were only two hospital wards where the poor mothers of Vienna could go for obstetrical care. And there it was expected that they would die in far greater numbers than the women from the middle and upper classes, who received better prenatal and obstetrical care.

On one charity ward, the cream of Vienna's obstetrical faculty provided free care for the indigent mothers as part of teaching medical students. These students would go regularly to the morgue, performing autopsies on women who had died after childbirth. In the other ward, Semmelweis was all alone. He was simply not well enough established to attract students. Semmelweis was too busy taking care of the indigent mothers single-handedly to perform any autopsies.

On the first ward, where students trafficked back and forth between the ward and the morgue, the mortality rate was three times higher than on Semmelweis's ward. As Semmelweis pored over the data, he hypothesized that the cause of the puerperal fever must be an infectious agent being spread from the bodies of the dead mothers to the delivering mothers by the hands of the students. Perhaps, he thought, if the students would scrub with soap and wash their hands with chlorine bleach after each dissection, the contagion could be interrupted and thousands of women's lives could be saved.

The medical establishment would have no part of Semmelweis's theories. Puerperal infection, they asserted, was just a natural risk of childbirth. Nothing could be done to stop it. Of course, in the twenty-first century, Semmelweis's idea is logical. It has made complete sense for a long time. One hundred fifty years earlier, however, his ideas were heresy. So denigrated was his suggestion that obstetrical faculty would threaten to flunk any student who participated in Semmelweis's proposed "alternative research."

But Semmelweis stubbornly refused to drop his theories or forsake the women who might be spared if his theory was correct. He invited a number of students onto his ward under one condition: they *must* wash their hands with soap and then rinse thoroughly in a chlorinated solution before examining *any* woman. When his instructions were followed, Semmelweis demonstrated, the mortality rate on his ward fell to 1.27 percent. The other ward's death rate was more than ten times higher, at 18.2 percent. What's more, from March to August 1848, not a single mother on Semmelweis's ward had died from puerperal fever.

The results were published. But Semmelweis was considered a troublesome upstart and he was simply thrown out of Austria and sent back to practice in Hungary. He had threatened one of the premier faculties of medicine in the world and paid the price by being banned forever. At home in Budapest, Semmelweis was undaunted. He repeated the experiment, successfully lowering the mortality rate to 0.15 percent in the St. Rochus Hospital, where he was now the head obstetrician.

Still, in Vienna, Berlin, and Prague, the puerperal infection death rate raged on at well over one hundred times the levels that Semmelweis had shown he could reproduce, repeatedly, in one hospital after another.

Semmelweis begged his fellow obstetricians to listen. Few would. Semmelweis himself eventually developed an infection in his right hand from a surgical mishap. He became devoted full-time to pleading for the universal adoption of his aseptic technique. Virtually no one in the medical establishment would listen to him. One of the most famous and revered physicians at that time, Rudolf Virchow, of Berlin, publicly rejected Semmelweis and his notions. The high and mighty of the surgical world called for an end to this madness about cleanliness and chlorinated decontamination. Semmelweis was run out of medicine.

The frustration and rejection took its toll on him. With his emotional and physical health shattered, Semmelweis had a nervous breakdown and was committed to a mental institution, where he died, broken and forgotten. The cause of his death was an overwhelming infection from puerperal fever in his hand. He literally died giving his life to the disease he had devoted himself to eradicating. His is one of the saddest stories in medicine. But I retell Semmelweis's story because it's an important reminder of just how reactionary the medical establishment can be to new, "alternative" therapies.

Alfred's mother began pouring pounds of shark cartilage into her son, coming to him every three or four hours with a milkshake— smelling as putrid as a fishmonger's stand—begging him, with tears in her eyes, to please drink the "shark shake."

It was obvious that Alfred was imploding. In its own way, his family was doing the same. I started making house calls to see them on the weekends. All over the kitchen counters were open bags of shark cartilage powder. I wrinkled my nose at the overpowering fishy odor. To my horror, I found out a bank had put a lien on the modest trailer where they lived. This was to ensure payment for all the debts Alfred's mother had run up to buy the cartilage.

Our spring break was coming up. Our family made plans to head north to spend a week skiing in Park City, outside Salt Lake City. By now Alfred was close to dying. He was admitted to the hospital. He'd become incontinent. Couldn't keep up with his fluids. He was gagging. Choking. Occasionally suffocating. He was spiraling downward. I didn't want to leave him now in the hands of strangers. So I made a fateful decision: I asked my family if I could cancel our vacation, stay in town, and take care of Alfred.

Of course, my wife and children understood. They could see why I wanted to tend to this child in his dying days. I had already persuaded myself to make this sacrifice. It might strike you as a noble act. It wasn't. It was one of the worst decisions I've ever made. My hubris was talking, making me think I was just too important for Alfred to entrust his care to anyone else. Even my own family had been dragged into participating in my martyrdom. The least I could have done was to send them on to Park City. But what good is a great sacrifice without an audience? I made a classic, rookie mistake. I should have gone skiing. Really. It sounds harsh. I should have known I was not indispensable—even for Alfred in his last moments.

Alfred died. He eased into death with a little morphine. On one side of the bed was his father praying to the Lord to take his son. On the other side, his mother begging God to take her life instead. The only substantive thing I did was to ensure that Alfred's dog could cuddle next to him in bed. The dog was smuggled into the hospital room in a large shopping bag. When a nurse discovered it, I wrote an order in the chart: "Dog to be at patient's bedside every nursing shift—no exceptions." This was at a time when a doctor's order still carried some weight. As soon as I proclaimed the dog to have medicinal potency, all objections from the nursing staff ceased. Alfred died with his beloved dog at his side.

The day after Alfred's funeral, I slept in. Later that morning, I sat looking out my window at the craggy summits of the Santa Catalina Mountains. I thought how good it was to just be alive. I was on my couch, gazing at the view, and turned to pick up my coffee cup. It was a turn of 30 degrees to one side at the most. Suddenly, my back buckled violently. It was nothing like my prior injury. I felt as if I'd been struck by lightning. I doubled over and fell to the floor. I lay there moaning, hardly daring to draw a breath. Electric shocks seemed to be going down both legs. Whereas before I had experienced a throbbing ache in my lower back, now it felt like something was tearing my very nerves out by the roots.

Janey came running. She tried to help me move my legs but it was impossible. The pain was too severe. She wanted to call 911 but I wouldn't let her. It would be unbearable if the paramedics tried to move me. She slipped two pain tablets onto the back of my tongue and held water to my lips so I could swallow them. I waited for them to take effect. A little later, I lay propped up against two pillows, with a blanket over me, trying to breathe deeply as the pain started to ease up.

I had no plan. I just lay on the floor praying the pain wouldn't come back, asking God for an answer—any answer.

About a minute or two later, there was a knock at the front door. I couldn't move, so I just yelled at whoever it was (UPS, the mailman, etc.) to walk in. The front door was open. Unexpectedly, a former student of mine walked through the front door. It was none other than Charlie Begay, a Navajo graduate student with whom I had prepared a syllabus on Native American medicine a year or two earlier. He had disappeared from my life after getting his master's degree in Public Health. Charlie walked in with a smile, as he always did. He spotted me and knelt down as though it were something he and I had practiced for years. I was embarrassed for him to see me on the living room floor, but he embraced me with great tenderness. He sat cross-legged, periodically holding my hand, as I explained what I thought was going on in my spine. I told him that I had undoubtedly herniated a disk. Gosh, I had a thousand crazy ideas at that moment. Cancer. Multiple sclerosis. I was swimming in panic.

"I've got to go now," Charlie said suddenly. "But I'll come back. And I'll bring help. Don't worry!" I had no idea what he meant.

So I was shocked when the doorbell rang hours later that evening. It was close to bedtime. My wife had helped me onto the couch earlier in the day and I had lain there all day, with two big pillows fluffed up under my knees. I had been taking pain relievers to take the edge off the pain and make it bearable. I was in no state for a social visit.

Charlie came into the living room, but this time he was not alone. He had brought a medicine man with him. I could tell what he was instantly. Over the years, I've had the honor of working with several medicine men. You can always spot them. They've got a certain power, a presence about them. There's a strange, enveloping warmth emanating from their hands too. I've only felt that warmth coming from the hands of sacred folks (and no, I don't have it).

Seeing the medicine man standing there was comforting and unnerving. I wasn't sure if the silver-haired, elegant gentleman spoke much English. If he did, he didn't use it. He spoke only to Charlie in Navajo. His commands were terse. Specific. Charlie listened and then turned to me:

"He says you must ask your whole family to come into this room. They will need to be here with you. And to help you." I was a little reluctant. It meant waking my youngest kids up. Seemed like a big fuss to rouse them. For what? But the medicine man was insistent. He wasn't going to budge until everyone was in the living room.

While my wife gathered the children, Charlie motioned toward the fireplace: "We will need to build a fire here. Is that okay?"

It was a warm evening for a fire but I reluctantly nodded my approval. The old man started a small fire, bringing the flames to life. He laid down fragrant sage and sweetgrass.

Charlie pulled a wooden chair in from the kitchen. He looked up toward the mountains, and I could tell he was squaring the chair so the old man would be properly seated in the north—the direction of wisdom and leadership. My three children sat on the couch, their eyes wide. The old shaman did his ministrations without so much as a nod in their direction. My oldest son, Josh, age thirteen, seemed intrigued.

Luke, my middle one, was only eight and seemed more apprehensive. My youngest, Tessa, three years old, was outright terrified. The children huddled together as the strange scents filled the air.

"You sit in this chair." Charlie motioned me toward a second chair, placed in the east.

How could I sit down? What was he talking about? I couldn't do that! I was in agony! "Come on, Charlie," I protested. "I can't even breathe without hurting. There's no way I'm getting up." I felt certain I must have herniated a lumbar disk or something. "I shouldn't move right now," I added.

"Get up," Charlie said icily. "It'll be okay. You must do it now. Right now." There was something insistent in his tone of voice that gave me a sense of dread. I wondered if something terrible would happen if I didn't get up. I did my best to make my way, hunched over, to the chair. The old man nodded his approval.

Charlie helped me into the chair. He whispered in my ear, "Do you think I would bring a great medicine man like Grandfather"—the term is used for any respected male elder—"here to hurt you?"

"No," I said. "Of course not. It's just that..."

"You've got to trust me. And him. If you can't, then he can't help you. You know that." He was quite firm with me. A bit of a role reversal.

I had to agree. Even though I'd been racked with spasms of pain and could not stand up straight all day long, I somehow managed to shuffle over to the chair with surprising ease and sit down.

Charlie ordered me to strip to the waist. The medicine man began fanning the small fire with an eagle feather fan. I closed my eyes and began to breathe deeply, trying to relax my tender back as much as possible. I listened carefully.

Charlie told me to surrender myself and not be afraid. "You are in the hands of a respected, beloved healer. Now, leave everything to him."

I nodded my assent.

The old man began a slow, deep-throated singing. The sound of his voice seemed to pass into the center of my body. I seemed to start vibrating in harmony with his chanting. He would sing and then blow into the fire, sending the sweet scent of sage into my lungs.

I felt his hands, like hot coals, on either side of my spine. I could feel love and kindness, pouring out from his being into mine. I had the sense he was somehow merging his hands inside my own body. And I suddenly became aware of an intuition that he might be putting himself at risk in doing so. He said something to Charlie.

"He says you must let go of someone. He has seen a boy in you, in his vision within you. A boy you love. He has already passed over to be with the Ancestors. But there is a tie, a string that holds him by his leg."

I had not said a word to Charlie or the shaman about Alfred's death. No one had. It was the farthest thing from my mind at that moment.

Charlie listened to the medicine man speak and then said, "My grandfather says that you have done this deed. You have tied this boy up, like a pony. You hobbled him by the leg, and you are holding his spirit back. You are clinging to him, yes? You have tied this boy by his ankle, and you are holding him fast. And you are holding him against his will. His ancestors call out to him but you stand in the way!" Charlie's voice was stern, almost outraged at this point, as he carried out his translation. "This boy's spirit is very angry with you. The boy's spirit is kicking you hard, to get loose, so he can be free. He wants to go. To join his ancestors in the spirit world. He's yelling at you to let him go."

The old man uttered a few more words. Charlie began translating again.

"Grandfather says that this young spirit wants to be finished with you!"

"I don't know what he's talking about," I said. But I did. I began to just sob. My shoulders started shaking uncontrollably. My children stared at me in complete astonishment. They had never seen me so distraught and vulnerable. It was a strange experience for them—for me too.

"Grandfather says that the boy is kicking so hard to get loose of your tight hold that he has kicked you in the back. That is why your spine hurts so much. He has kicked you, like a mule would kick to get free of a coyote that holds on to his leg."

The medicine man breathed deeply into the fire. The smoke rose into the air; warmth from his hands and the scent of the sage seemed to be circulating inside my abdominal cavity now. I was crying uncontrollably. Because deep inside I felt ashamed of myself for holding on to Alfred so tightly.

"Grandfather says that if you do not let go of this boy's spirit soon, it will just kill you. It will keep kicking at you till you are dead—that is how badly it desires to be rid of you."

"I will let go. I will let go!" I sobbed. I felt helpless. I continued crying out loudly. Janey jumped up to come to my aid. Charlie held up his hand to check her advance.

"No," he admonished. "You must stay seated and pray for your husband! Do not get up! Do not interfere or the spirit of this boy may strike out at you. Or," he added ominously, as he looked over at my three children seated in a row, "one of your children. He could snatch its soul as retribution. And then the boy would roam the earth as the living dead. Sit down!" he ordered.

Janey returned to the safety of the couch and put her arm around our youngest as if to protect her.

I was now inexplicably dripping in perspiration. I didn't feel unusually warm or febrile, but rivulets of sweat were running down my torso and soaking the waistband of my pants. I was sweating as hard as I was sobbing. I remember watching the waistband of my pants turning dark before my eyes with the liquid running down me like a fountain.

The medicine man talked to Charlie in Navajo. His voice was chopped, stern. Charlie translated: "You must send this boy away now...forever. He's very angry because he feels you are trying to turn him into a ghost. You must tell him to go away. To leave you forever. Now!" he barked, and he clapped his hands.

I did. My voice was husky from crying but I said aloud, "Alfred, I'm sorry. Go. Get away. Get out! Get out of my life!" I yelled with all the power I could summon, "Now! Go! Now!"

The shaman continued exhaling his warm breath against my lower back. I suddenly became quite calm. The pain in my back started fading. The pain became an ache that was no longer of any concern. The shaman fluttered an eagle fan all about my head and body. There was a gentle quality about the ruffling of the feathers, almost like little kisses. When it was all over, he said some clipped words to Charlie.

"The boy's spirit has gone. The spirit is grateful that you came to your senses. It will not trouble you any longer. Grandfather will prepare a bundle of herbs for you. You should make a tea from this each morning and drink it."

The old man interjected a few more words.

"Grandfather says you should get up each morning as the sun is rising and drink the tea facing eastward. The tea will restore your strength. He is finished now. It is over."

"Tell Grandfather that I am grateful for his care and...his love." Charlie translated. The old man smiled at me and then returned to wrapping up his feather fan with great care. I put my shirt back on, amazed at the amount of sweat that had poured out of me. Charlie admonished me to drink plenty of water and stay away from caffeine for a day or two.

I pulled him aside and asked him if it was appropriate to pay the shaman for his services. Charlie leaned over close to my ear and whispered, "Yes, it's a good thing to pay him. Pay him whatever you wish, but fifty dollars is good. Also, if you have tobacco in the house, that is a traditional gift. And you must cook him a meal so he can eat his fill before he departs."

"Cook him a meal? How? It's eleven-thirty at night!" I asked, trying not to raise my voice.

"You are standing here arguing with me? Don't you feel better?"

He was right. I was standing perfectly straight. I hadn't even been aware of how much better I felt. I sensed how dangerous my conflicting emotions about holding on to Alfred had become. I'm convinced the old medicine man saved my life.

"No, I'm grateful. It's just real late for a dinner. The kids have already eaten, and I have no idea what's in the house, that's all."

"I know that Grandfather came as soon as he could, no matter what time it was."

"Okay. Will spaghetti do?"

"Yes, John loves Italian." It was the first time Charlie had mentioned his name.

So the whole family cooked a giant pot of spaghetti. I made meatballs with marinara sauce with fresh crushed garlic. The kids helped make crispy garlic bread. We were all in great spirits. I felt physically so much better. It was if some dark cloud were gone from our lives. I was going to put out a bottle of Chianti, but Charlie waved it away, telling me politely that alcohol cannot come close to a medicine man when he is in a holy state like the one John had entered on my behalf. Charlie confirmed my impressions that John had, in fact, endangered a part of his own soul to help heal my own. He had been willing to put himself at risk for me, his patient.

This is the one critical difference between healing and just practicing medicine. Healing requires that physician and patient enter into partnership, facing dangers together. Two lives at risk! Medicine was not meant to be a mechanical transaction. It's a spiritual quest, putting your own soul on the line, along with the patient's.

Even though it was nearly midnight, everyone was famished. John's smile was broad and wonderful. He never said a word to me, but I got the clear impression that he was quite pleased with me, that he knew what was going through my head. He knew that gathering the requisite insights was a difficult, personal journey for any of us who wish to become healers.

As he stood up to leave, I handed him a bundle of old pipe tobacco I had lying around, fifty dollars, and a bright, new Pendleton blanket as a gift. I had the blanket as an early Christmas present for my brother, but the image of it suddenly jumped into my head, and I went down to the bedroom closet and pulled it off the shelf. John ran his hand carefully along the pile of the blanket. He smiled and then put his hand on my shoulder and embraced me. He also touched my children's heads—a gesture of blessing to each of them. Then John left. I have not seen him or heard of him since. Charlie never mentioned another word about him. I have been around Native Americans enough to know better than to ask too. As one of my fellow physicians once observed, "Indians are in on something that we Anglos don't get."

Alfred's parents divorced soon after his death. Whatever had held the family together was gone—a common occurrence in families that are wrestling with cancer or lose a loved one. Cancer hurts whole families, rarely just one member of it. In some cases, it can bring a family together and cement their sense of being connected to one another. In other cases the ties are too badly strained to survive.

Each year, a day or two ahead of Alfred's birthday, a card arrives addressed to me, in care of the Brain Research Laboratory. It is left tucked under the edge of the bronze plaque on the lab door. No one knows how it gets there. No one has ever seen anyone come or go. The section of the building is under tight security, so it would normally take some doing to get to the lab. Nobody can identify the simple handwriting with any of the correspondence from Alfred's parents or siblings. But for over a decade, the card is always there on time. The message each year inside the card is always the same: "Alfred, you are with us always."

I have never missed a vacation after that year with Alfred. I became more sparing about my how much of my own heart I could safely give to a patient under my care. I still struggle with that one, because I am keenly aware that a real healer, a powerful healer, must have enough power and skill to put part of himself at risk but still guarantee the safety of the patient and himself. A healer has to be committed but completely unattached, the way John was that night with me.

I've grown humbler now. I've come to realize that the sheer intensity of my own emotions cannot save another person, and under certain circumstances, it can actually become dangerous. In the early twentieth century, Walter B. Cannon, a famous Harvard physiologist, became fascinated with how apparently young men and women could die quite unexpectedly after a curse had been placed upon them. The so-called "voodoo death" occurred, he believed, because the cursed individual's emotions were so powerful that they literally killed the body. He commented that each voodoo death had to be understood as an individual dying because of strongly held beliefs.

It was my own guilt over losing Alfred with which the shaman had to wrestle. I had spent so much emotional energy over Alfred that I had created a malevolent spirit of enormous strength out of my own feelings. The shaman had the skill and strength to help me confront my monster. He showed me that the master healer is involved but, at the same time, totally disconnected, impeccably objective about what he must do.

I'm convinced that our personal feelings have enormous impact on our health. I believe that negative feelings—anger, guilt, hatred, resentment, regret, envy—are quite dangerous emotional energies, because they are destructive to the individual that harbors them. So Cannon's voodoo death was really the beginning of a scientific inquiry into today what has become the field of psychoneuroimmunology—the study of how emotions interact within the body through the mind.

The mind is the greatest secret in all of medicine. John's great shamanic gift was this: You cannot heal if you cannot feel. Healing isn't from the brain but the soul. You've got to look for it in the right places, armed with the correct attitude. Without impeccability, there is no healing power.

Eleven

Thread of Hope

Life is God's novel. Let Him write it.

Isaac Bashevis Singer

ndrew Weil is my friend. To many of you who know him, it is no surprise that I sought him out as a healer nearly fifteen years ago. Andy is also a visionary in modern-day American medicine. *Newsweek* magazine featured him on the cover with a question: "Will this man change the face of American medicine?"

For me, the answer is simply: yes. He already has! When no one was willing to consider combining alternative medicine with mainstream (also known as allopathic) medicine, Andy coined the term "integrative medicine." He believes one type of medical therapy is not necessarily exclusive of another school or style. Two types of therapy can complement each other. The physical and spiritual aspects of medicine do not need to be seen as opposite or antagonistic. Andy showed me that even as a surgeon, I could embrace medicine as both a spiritual and a scientific quest.

Andy taught me to never be afraid of "hope" as an integral ingredient of any therapeutic approach. He asserts there is no such thing as "false hope." Hope is simply the desire to prevail, to survive, and to win against overwhelming odds.

I've often heard colleagues withholding a new form of treatment because "the drug is experimental" and "I don't want to give the patient any false hopes." Andy taught me to take exception to such statements—

as an individual and as a physician. Too many physicians focus on the sterile, scientific nihilism that banishes hope, forbids it. Physicians and surgeons have been taught how *not* to see the miraculous and magical. We've become overcome by a scientific cynicism that precludes hope manifesting itself in our patients' lives—even in our own life. Physicians are trained to see the obvious, the concrete. Manifestations of the divine and the sacred are considered intrinsically suspect.

I have had to learn a great deal about hope. It was not a subject matter taught in medical school or residency. Hope is just not on the curriculum. So I learned about it the hard way—by killing it. Then I found out that hope is as fundamental a tool to any surgeon as a scalpel.

Hope manifested itself clearly for me in two different scenarios. Both involved patients under my care. They both also became my friends. One was a truck driver and the other a famous medical researcher. I couldn't have asked for two more different teachers—from different walks of life or segments of society. Together, they shared wonderful and humbling experiences with me.

Donald brought home the first, terrible lesson on hope. He was twenty-three years old when I met him. He'd been a typical small-town hero. High school quarterback. He didn't have the grades or the background to believe college was within his grasp. Instead, he went into the family's trucking business. It was run by his parents out of a depot in Flagstaff, Arizona. He didn't love driving trucks, but it pleased his old man to see him behind the wheel of the big rigs. His mom was happy just to hail her son on the CB radio as he sped along I-17 toward home. His handle was "Fly Fisherman."

Fly-fishing was Donald's passion. Although he was first taught by his dad, Donald quickly surpassed him. In Coconino National Forest, where there are streams galore, he soon became one of the best. Since Arizona is largely desert, if you gain respect as a fisherman in northern Arizona, you've earned a statewide reputation.

Donald kept a fly-tying jig in his truck so he could turn out new flies whenever he pulled off the road to rest or was caught in a traffic jam. He made so many flies, he couldn't use them all. At first, he just gave them away to folks in the veterans' home outside the nearby town of Prescott. Soon the vets started ordering flies to give to relatives and friends, and eventually it became a little business on the side. It was a big deal for Donald when two of the most prestigious fly-fishing firms in the country decided to offer his flies in their mail order catalogs. To most of the world, he was just a truck driver. But to the fly-fishing world, he was becoming the reclusive master of Flagstaff who made those incredible one-of-a-kind flies. At twenty-three, he'd become an underground legend. It tickled him to be greeted at the odd bait-and-tackle store in Idaho or Montana like a visiting celebrity.

One day in October 1994, while teaching his youngest nephew to catch cutthroat trout in Oak Creek Canyon, a few miles outside of Sedona, Donald noticed that he couldn't cast a fly into the pools with his usual expertise. In fact, his nephew commented on how many flies Donald was landing in the rocks and trees. When Donald's mom was told what happened, she joked that at his current selling prices, her son had lost more than three hundred dollars in one afternoon! Until that day, Donald had not lost a single fly in years.

Donald suspected something was up. He later told me he tossed and turned all that night. The next morning he woke up with a pounding headache, and that soon became a daily event. Often the headaches came on with nausea so severe that it could make him skip his mother's home-cooked biscuits. A week after the fly-fishing disaster, he noticed that the sunlight on the road and reflection off the windshield had started bothering him. In fact, he stopped in Las Vegas and bought a second pair of sunglasses, which he wore on top of his original pair to cut down on the glare. He began taking Tylenol around the clock. Ten days later, on a job in Eugene, Oregon, he ran his truck into a parked station wagon. Up until that moment he had never even so much as scratched his rig. Something was seriously wrong.

Donald called his doctor on the way home. At that time, Flagstaff was still a small town, where you would just call up your doctor (who had probably known you all your life) and you'd be instructed to come right in. Buck McComb had taken care of Donald through a host of football injuries, including a couple of dramatic concussions. He knew Donald was a stoic fellow—not the sort to complain—so he told Donald to drive straight over to his office.

Nothing could have prepared him for the transformation that showed up at the door. For two weeks Donald had barely been able to keep food down. He had lost nearly twenty pounds. The headaches woke him incessantly during the night, and he was desperately sleep-deprived. With huge, dark circles under his eyes, and holding on to the walls to steady himself, he looked as though he was coming off a bender. But Dr. McComb knew better: Donald didn't drink.

Dr. McComb drove Donald straight to the emergency room at Flagstaff Medical Center and examined him there while waiting for a CT scan. On the basis of the physical alone, it was clear something was dreadfully wrong. For one thing, nearly half of Donald's visual field was gone. That was the reason he had plowed into the parked car. He had never even seen it.

You may wonder: How can you lose half your vision and not even know it? If you think about it, however, as you read these words, you can't see anything behind your head. Now, hold your arms out and swing them around from the front toward the back. You will reach a point on the side when your hands are no longer visible. In medical terms, they now lie outside your visual field.

But the brain does something quite elegant with visual fields. Although we see only a small part of the world around us at any one moment, we have an inner sense of it being whole and complete. For instance, imagine that you are focusing on a spot on the wall ahead of you. As you continue to look straight at it, you will notice that you can actually see a good deal around the periphery of that spot. You have a sense that you are seeing the whole room. But you are actually seeing only what is in your visual field. In fact, if it were possible to do so in complete silence, someone could dismantle everything outside your visual field, and you would be stunned to discover you might, for example, actually be standing out under a tree or in a parking lot. The brain fools us into thinking we are seeing the world around us when we actually can only visualize one small part of it at a time.

The brain compensates so well for change that you may not even be cognizant of it. Your visual field could be gradually downsized, for instance, and you might not know it for quite some time. That's what happened to Donald. His visual world had diminished by more than half. That's also why he'd had such a terrible time casting his flies a few weeks earlier.

When Dr. McComb had the CT scan images in hand, all Donald's symptoms made sense. There was a tumor in the back of the brain— in the occipital lobe, where visual function occurs. It was the size of a peach and was causing a significant amount of swelling and pressure on the brain. That pressure was producing the headaches and the nausea and vomiting. The photophobia (in Latin, it means "scared of light" but actually refers to the patient's need to reduce incoming bright light) also indicated significant buildup of pressure inside his brain.

It was clear to Dr. McComb that Donald had a life-threatening problem. He instructed the family to pack Donald up and drive him down to the University Medical Center in Tucson. I finally got the call and spread the word to our team to get ready for Donald's arrival.

The University of Arizona is blessed with a marvelous telemedicine center (telemedicine enables doctors and patients to confer with each other at a distance), so I was able to talk through a video image hookup with Buck. I reviewed all the findings and actually looked at the CT scans with them as Donald's family was preparing to leave. I asked Buck if he had discussed the findings with the family. He had told them it looked like a brain tumor and that the surgery was too complex for them to do up there. They wanted to go to Tucson. They wanted everything done.

"Do they know it might be malignant?" I asked.

"Nope. I didn't go into any of that," he answered.

Fine. That was going to be my job.

Donald arrived about six hours later. I met the family as they were trudging through the door of our busy emergency room. My nurse, Darlene, had already made all the arrangements to have Donald admitted to the hospital. All his patient information had been entered into the computer. He could go right back to an examination room, lie down on a gurney, and get a little rest. I could see the stress in their faces.

Over the two decades I've been doing brain tumor surgery, I've been impressed by the disproportionate number of sweet, kind people stricken with this tragic condition. I don't espouse the theory that God visits this horrific disease only on those who can handle it. But I have wondered if being diagnosed with a tumor doesn't somehow enlighten these patients. The majority possess an almost otherworldly, saintly quality. It's like a divine presence has made itself manifest to them, more tangible and visible. So it was with Donald. He immediately began thanking me and was worried that he had taken up too much of my time. He seemed more intent on getting his parents settled in for the night near the medical center than having everyone focus on his brain tumor.

"Don't you worry. Your mom and I will stay in the RV right out in the parking lot. That way we'll be right there if you need us," his father pronounced formally. He looked up at me almost sheepishly. "You know the doctors might need us for something, for information or something like that." He wanted to stay as close as he could to his son right now.

Over the next twenty-four hours, we ran all the tests, getting ourselves ready for surgery. The following day Donald was anesthetized in the operating room. After six hours of surgery, the tumor was removed. He made an excellent recovery and was eating breakfast the morning after. He was discharged two days later. The visual field cut—the lost area of his vision—however, was permanent. The tumor had invaded that whole area of the left visual cortex, so when we dissected out the malignant nest of cells, that area of the brain was also removed. But the headaches disappeared as soon as the tumor was gone.

The plan was to bring him back in a week to remove the surgical stitches. In the meantime, we took the tumor specimen to our neuro-oncology laboratory, where the research technicians under Larry, our lab director, tried to learn everything they could about how the tumor was behaving. What they learned was chilling.

In the brain, a malignant tumor is one whose cells have the capacity to divide, reproduce, and invade the brain's own tissue. One measure of the aggressiveness of a tumor is a characteristic called the mitotic index, or MI. The MI tells a cell biologist what fraction of cells within a tumor are dividing at that moment. Although most cancers grow rapidly, only a very small fraction of their cells are reproducing at an instant. Normally, even very aggressive tumors are relatively inefficient and will have an MI of 7 to 15 percent (15 percent is considered very high).

I got a call from Larry.

"You know this tumor you sent down to us?" he asked.

"The one we took out of the kid from Flagstaff?"

"Yep, that's the one."

"Well, what about it?"

"You aren't going to believe it, but that damn thing has an MI of 92!"

"That's ridiculous. No one can have a tumor that divides that fast. There's gotta be something wrong with the lab equipment," I said.

"Nope. I've run it four separate times on four separate specimens with four different technicians. It really is 92 percent. This tumor is dividing faster than any cell line I've seen in twenty years of cell biology."

My brain went right to work. I thought perhaps the high mitotic index would at least give me some kind of edge. "Well, is that something we can exploit?" I asked. "You know what I mean? If it's growing so fast, then won't all those cells be more susceptible to radiation and chemotherapy because so few will be lying low and not dividing? Only 8 percent will be dormant."

One thing I've learned over the years is that every tumor is different. Even though the pathologists group tumors by the same name, like glioblastoma multiforme (GBM for short), it's just a label. Like hearing someone's name is Bill. What does that tell you? The label is not the thing it describes. Donald's tumor was clearly a different type of glioblastoma multiforme from any we'd ever seen before in our laboratory.

Every tumor is nature's experiment of one. We have to watch the experiment unfold. We can't make assumptions just because the last five tumors of this type behaved a certain way. This new one might not live by the same rules. We can't ignore the variability that nature introduces into everything: are any two oak trees or snowflakes the same? Each tumor is a unique representative of its class or histological grade, presenting individual traits and susceptibility. So in the tumor's individuality, hope can blossom. Because we can exploit the unique weaknesses of each tumor, we must not settle into a cynicism that says: none of these tumors do well, so why go after them? What if the very next tumor holds the secret, the key, to the discovery that will open a new, potent avenue of therapy? We'd never even notice if we didn't approach each tumor with hope and a genuine respect for the diversity of tumor biology.

When Donald returned to have his stitches out, I shared with him the unique characteristics Larry had discovered about his tumor. He asked me, understandably, if this was good news or bad? I said honestly I didn't know. On the one hand, a tumor that could actually attain such alarming rates of cell division and reproduction was formidable. However, this could also provide a target-rich environment (in military parlance). These cells could prove very susceptible to the effects of both radiation and chemotherapy. Both types of treatment are really aimed at the vulnerable stages when cells reproduce and must replicate their DNA, the genetic code in their chromosomes.

A broad grin broke out on Donald's face. "Boy, I like the sound of that! Let's get those cells! Let's just hammer them!" He pounded his fist into his hand for emphasis. "When do we get started?" he asked.

"Next week," I answered.

"Isn't that too much time to not be doing anything?"

I hadn't thought of that. A week one way or the other doesn't really matter when you're dealing with the average tumor, with a mitotic index of 4 or 8 percent. But this was 92!

"I think you might be right. This tumor shouldn't wait. Normally we would give you an extra week to get over the effects of surgery and to be sure the wound is healed, but your incision is looking fine."

"I'm as strong as a bull, doc. You'll see."

What followed was six weeks of nonstop radiation therapy delivered every single day. I saw Donald lose his hair. I saw the grinding fatigue set in. The circles beneath his eyes. Not once did he complain or lose his enthusiasm. As soon as the radiation was finished, we launched into an aggressive regimen of intravenous chemotherapy for another six weeks. It was a marathon. Had Donald not been so young and strong, he could never have tolerated all of it. But he did splendidly, and the tumor really responded. Clearly the high rate of cell division made his tumor exquisitely susceptible to all the treatments, especially since they were literally being heaped upon one another. I pictured the filaments of Donald's tumor, standing like so many thousands of soldiers, being mowed down by this blistering barrage of cannon fire, followed by a chemotherapeutic cavalry assault. I saw the ranks of DNA falling back, being hit again by another salvo, falling back again. Each time the group shrank in number and huddled together as the onslaught continued.

Donald's first CT scans after completion of the three-month blitzkrieg looked pristine. There was an obvious resection cavity where we had removed the tumor. Its edges were smooth and there was no enhancement. This meant that intravenous contrast dye was not being absorbed in this area. A very good sign. His neurological examination had not changed one bit, and his hair was even starting to grow back— although it was thinner and fuzzier.

I reconvened with Donald and his family in our outpatient clinic and we tried to lay out some more strategy. I explained that GBMs are almost never cured. In fact, there was one Scandinavian study performed to determine what the chances were of being a long-term survivor. Sweden has an excellent medical care system, entirely socialized. Every patient diagnosed with a GBM is entered in a national data registry. The government can follow every patient from diagnosis to death. They tracked five thousand patients to see how many were still alive five years after their tumors had been diagnosed. The numbers were dismal: only five out of five thousand patients with GBM had survived five years or more. The odds of being a long-term survivor were exactly one in a thousand!

I may have to share this information with every patient at some point in the course of the illness, but with two caveats. First, the Swedish study was done before really aggressive multimodality therapies were available. We're still unprepared to assess the impact these strategies will have on long-term survival. Second, I have six patients who are alive and well at more than five years (I'll get to that) out from diagnosis. And I did not have six thousand patients under my care over that period of time. So exceptions clearly exist to these statistical findings.

But the bottom line is that GBMs are usually incurable. You never get to stop the treatments. We knew—and I made sure Donald was onboard—the only way to hold this tumor at bay was to keep pounding away at it. So Donald was put back on another three rounds of chemotherapy. We also hit the center of the tumor cavity with the intense single-fraction radiation of "radiosurgery." This treatment delivers a staggering amount of radiation just to the rind, or shell, where the tumor cells are most likely to grow back. With each successive blow, Donald's body would seem to shudder a little: a drop in cell counts, a bout of pneumonia, a blood clot in his left leg. Always he would rebound. He would come back the same, smiling, optimistic Donald.

One day about a year into this odyssey, Donald asked me if he could stay after his parents left and talk privately with me. I've learned that when a patient or a family member pulls you aside, it will usually be an important conversation. Donald closed the door to the exam room and leaned close to me, almost whispering:

"Doc, it's about this tumor. I know what you've been tellin' me. I understand there's a chance I might not beat this thing, that it could grow back or something in a way that nothing could kill it. I figure this tumor's just like any other wild creature that gets hunted over and over. If it survives, it's because it's getting smarter and smarter. Every time you shoot, it gets more and more savvy until it's too smart to kill."

There was some real truth in what Donald said. Tumor cells do, in fact, mutate to become more and more resistant to radiation, to chemotherapy, and even surgical resection. I nodded my head affirmatively to what Donald was saying.

"So I guess there might come a time," he continued, "when the tumor might be draggin' me down. Makin' it so I am weak or can't walk straight. Or maybe makin' me loopy, wacky."

Tears welled up in his eyes. "I...I just don't want my mom to have to see me like that. I don't want her takin' care of me in that shape. So if things are headin' south for me, I want you to tell me when it's time to go fishin', if you know what I mean. That's real important to me. Just tell me to head out and go fishin'. You understand?" he asked.

He looked right at me. "Promise me, doc, you'll let me know real straight when it's time for me to give up and go fishin', okay?"

"I promise. I give you my word that I'll let you know...if it comes to that," I said.

"Well, sure! Hell, I'm not givin' up on this tumor. You know me better'n that, don't you?" Donald answered back.

All of a sudden, his face brightened. He smiled. The energy flowed back into his face. His eyes cleared and regained their light composure. He and I wouldn't have to speak about this conversation again. It was always replaying in the back of our minds. I knew I would live up to my pledge.

For the second year, Donald's scans appeared reasonably dormant. The tumor seemed to be in remission. We had wiped Donald out with the chemotherapy. But champion that he was, he rallied and was strong enough to go fishing and even elk hunting along the rugged Mogollon Plateau country of northern Arizona. He always brought me a trout or a choice cut from the elk loin, or a huge ponderosa pine cone—a souvenir from each adventure. Once he brought me a shed antler from a mule deer. I had a small shelf in one corner of my office where I collected these mementos. Each time I added to the collection it was another con-crete reminder of Donald's undaunted determination to stay alive.

In the third year, however, the tumor did return. With a vengeance. It was like a creature that had been wounded, had gotten up, and was now stalking him. Enraged, it hunted him down. A routine scan sud-denly showed the tumor was growing rapidly. It had not only returned in the resection cavity but was now moving rapidly along several white-matter tracts to get to other parts of the brain. It had also started invad-ing the sides of the lateral ventricle.

Ventricles are spaces inside of the brain filled with a clear, watery fluid called cerebrospinal fluid, or CSF. CSF bathes the inside of the entire brain, circulating continuously from the center, down around the spinal cord, then back up over the outside surface of the brain before draining into the venous circulation along the inside of the skull. When a GBM is growing in the ventricle, the tumor is free to shed cells into the stream of CSF flowing through the ventricles. It can gain access to virtually any portion of the brain or spinal cord that is bathed in CSF. I could already see a few seedling nodules forming like tiny pearls at dif-ferent spots in the CSF pathway. As Donald had pointed out, this tumor had become very savvy. It was spreading throughout the brain, going to locations that could not be irradiated or would not receive a good distri-bution of chemotherapy.

I reviewed the scans with Donald and his parents. We would need to start a new line of aggressive therapy. We also decided to resect as much of the solid tumor as we could, because it was going to crush the adja-cent normal brain. So once again, I would have to go back into Don-ald's brain and attack the tumor surgically. It would be more difficult this time because of scar tissue. Also, the tumor was developing a very intense blood supply by scavenging blood vessels belonging to normal brain tissue. It was a devastating view of a histologically ruthless tumor. Donald, however, seemed to find new reserves of strength. His stamina was awe-inspiring. Following surgery, he threw himself with total con-centration into the next round of energy-depleting chemotherapy.

Within three months, the tumor's spread was clogging the flow through the ventricles. In the early hours of the Saturday after Thanksgiving, Donald's parents brought him into the ER. They had found him comatose in bed. I rushed to the Medical Center while an emergent CT scan was obtained. It showed that during the night one of the ventricles had become completely obstructed and had swelled up to three times its normal size. It was putting so much pressure on Donald's brain stem that he had sunk into a coma.

I looked at him. I remembered how much he had endured. I couldn't help but wonder: Would it be so terrible to just let him slip off to sleep forever? My next thought was: Who was I to make such a decision for another human being? Who was I to think that life was too difficult, or too much of a struggle for someone else? It was not my place to make that decision, and besides, I had made a pledge to Donald—albeit a difficult one now to keep.

I talked things over with Donald's parents. His mother was weeping so desperately I couldn't make out half of what she said. I did get that she was pleading with me, begging me to do anything, everything to save her boy. His father nodded sadly, and we made the decision to take Donald to the operating room and relieve the obstruction.

The operation took an hour and a half. I installed a device called a ventriculoperitoneal shunt, which bypasses the obstruction and dumps the excessive fluid in the abdomen, where it can be easily absorbed by the walls of the gut. By the end of the surgery, Donald was wide awake. He was back as bright as a brand-new penny.

Because the tumor was still growing, we turned to more experimental, far-out chemotherapies. The world of brain tumors is a very small one, even on the global scale. All the major research groups worldwide are in constant contact over the Internet sharing the latest research developments and chemotherapy protocols. We were well hooked up, and for a while, anyway, Donald seemed to be responding to a new experimental agent.

Over the next three months, he rallied. The shunt was keeping him out of life-threatening danger. In the spring, though—on April Fools' Day, actually—the shunt malfunctioned. Donald sank into a coma again and was once again rushed to the hospital. Our operating team was standing by. I took a quick CT scan to confirm that the shunt had become blocked, and we went back to the surgical suite and revised it. It was completely blocked—tumor cells were growing inside it!

The day after surgery, Donald was already eating and asking to go home. I knew we could discharge him the next morning. I also knew it was time to keep my word: It was time to go fishing.

I waited until all the residents and nurses had finished their usual flurry of morning rounds and paperwork. Donald was sitting up in bed, ready to leave, in his T-shirt and sweatpants. He had a bulky dressing where we had reopened his incisions to install the latest shunt. He looked like a poor caricature of a turbaned genie.

I poked my head around the corner of the curtain near the bed. "Hey, Donald. I need to talk for a sec."

"Sure. What's up?"

I explained about the shunt. I told him it was only a matter of time—maybe weeks or even days—until the shunt clogged again and we would be right back where we started. I explained that the tumor was now seeding quickly throughout the cerebrospinal fluid.

He stared at me blankly. At first, I thought maybe it was just grim resignation. And then it dawned on me: He didn't realize it was over! He didn't know he was dying! I sat down on the end of the bed. I looked him straight in the eye. "Donald, you remember once you asked me to tell you straight when it was time to go fishing?" I asked.

He nodded and looked down at his feet.

"Well, it is time. Now, Donald." My voice sounded almost harsh.

He didn't look up. He just sat there with his head bowed. I could see the tears falling onto his lap. I stayed there awhile. I knew the message had hit home.

After a few minutes of silence, I asked, "Hey, is there anything you need right now, buddy?" It seemed inappropriately upbeat, but I felt helpless.

Donald just shook his head no. I left the room quietly.

By the time he was discharged, a couple of hours later, he was a completely beaten young man. His eyes had lost their brightness. The energy that had sustained him—all of us, really—throughout his ordeal was gone.

I scheduled a follow-up appointment for one week so I could check the shunt's function. I went over the usual discharge and wound-healing instructions, but Donald wasn't listening. I decided to repeat it all to his mom, just so there would be another set of attentive ears. Donald solemnly hugged each of the nurses and then all the residents. Finally he hugged me and pressed a beautiful, red and green, fuzzy, custom-made mayfly and hook into my hand: "This is just what you'd be needing this time of year for trout. They'll come right up to the surface and bite hard...and fast. They're real hungry right now." He smiled.

In retrospect, I should have understood what was really going on.

The next morning Donald's mother called me. She was sobbing. Donald had expired during the night. He was gone.

I am convinced Donald died that night because the hope that had sustained him was taken away. When I had said it was "time to go fishing," I mistakenly cut the thin thread of hope that had kept him alive and aloft. He didn't die directly from his tumor. Instead, he died from despair. He died from my inadvertent disregard for what was really keeping him alive. In a way, I had finally committed my own form of voodoo death. I was learning. The hard way.

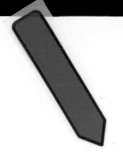

Singing in the Brain

*I know what the great cure is: it is to give up, to relinquish, to surrender, so that
our little hearts may beat in unison with the great heart of the world.*

HENRY MILLER

M y second story about hope also involved a brain tumor. In one of
my own colleagues. It provided me with one of my most public
failures in my career as a neurosurgeon.

Sidney "Sy" Sonnenberg was one of the outstanding Alzheimer's disease specialists in the country. He had helped discover balled-up proteins, called neurofibrillary tangles. The amount of these tangles in the brain appeared to correlate closely with both the severity and onset of Alzheimer's. His idea was simple and brilliant: as the patient's brain cells became clogged with this dysfunctional protein, it led to widespread cognitive disorder and dementia. His theories paved the way for nearly two decades of therapy designed at forestalling or reversing Alzheimer's disease.

Sy had been asked to preside over a prestigious Pan-Asian conference on Alzheimer's research and was on his way to the meeting in Auckland, New Zealand. Sitting in his business-class seat, enjoying a cocktail, he turned to his wife, Joanne, with a sudden look of consternation on his face. She asked him what was wrong. But he didn't answer. He just stared at her. He looked confused and lost.

"Joanne, I forgot how to ask for peanuts." He seemed mystified.

"You want peanuts?" she asked, almost annoyed. "I'll get you some peanuts."

"No," said Sy softly. "I forgot how to ask for them. I couldn't make the words, find the words. They wouldn't come out."

Suddenly Joanne was worried. Sy reassured her. Whatever had occurred seemed to have vanished as suddenly as it had appeared. But deep down, he wondered if he'd just experienced a transient ischemic attack (TIA), a kind of ministroke caused by a small blood clot. Of course, he didn't say anything to Joanne. But he did swallow two aspirin—just in case. And he continued to take aspirin for the next few days, hoping it would keep any potential stroke from developing.

There were no more episodes—as far as anyone knew—until the final day of the conference, when he was awarded the Larson Award for his pioneering work in the pathological diagnosis of Alzheimer's. He delivered the keynote address. For an hour the audience was mesmerized by the brilliance of his data and his theories about cortical dementia—when neurons stop participating in rich cortical circuits and cognitive function ebbs away. During the speech, Sy experienced several more spells of word-finding difficulty, each lasting a split second and only perceptible as a pause or a breath. No one noticed a thing. Except Sy. He knew the truth. At least three times during the lecture, his brain had scrambled furiously for the right word. Sy knew something was going terribly wrong with his brain.

He came off the podium to thundering applause and a standing ovation and hurried over to Joanne.

"It happened again," he whispered to her.

"What?"

"The words. They stopped coming."

"You mean during your speech? I listened to it. You never stumbled or stammered."

"No, you couldn't hear it. But I sure as hell knew it. Let's go home."

Twenty-four hours later, Sy and Joanne were together in my office, huddled next to me over his MRI scans. There was no evidence of a

stroke, and studies of the arteries in his neck and skull showed no significant underlying issues. But something else was there. Something
worse than any TIA. The scan revealed a large tumor in the junction of
the temporal and parietal lobes underlying the area where speech origi-
nates. One look and Sy knew. One look at my face and Joanne knew. It
was a glioblastoma multiforme—the dreaded GBM.

Treating Sy was more difficult for me than with a routine patient.
He knew more about cognitive dysfunction and more about the brain
specifically than I did—more than almost anyone alive. He knew about
GBMs' aggressive behavior. He knew before I could get the words out
that he had a terrible prognosis. And he knew he was going to need a
surgeon to operate.

"What do you want to do, Sy? You want me to call Bobby Winston
in San Francisco?"

Bobby was probably the most famous glioma surgeon in the United
States at the time. "If you want him to operate, I'll get him on the phone.
We can have you up there tomorrow."

"No, you do it," Sy said.

"You sure? I have no problem sending you to San Francisco."

"I'm sure. I want you to do it." He gave a snort of laughter. "You
won't get creative. Take a little more here or there." Then he got serious.
"Joanne and I have decided. You do the surgery tomorrow."

Sy's tone was almost an order. I booked the operating room for the
next morning and spent most of that evening mapping the tumor at my
computer workstation. The tumor seemed to reach right up to, if not
into, the speech area. Miraculously, however, Sy hadn't had more serious speech problems. And that was what worried me.

The tumor had grown into his speech area without disturbing very
much. From Sy's perspective, that was great. But for me, it was para-
doxically dreadful. I could end up making things worse. The risk was
I might actually destroy his speech capacity in the process of removing
the tumor. Briefly, perversely, I wished the tumor had done more damage so the stakes of the surgery would not be so high.

I went over the scans again. This area is high-priced real estate, as neurosurgeons say. Especially on the dominant left side. I returned to the computer image of the tumor. It was almost surreal. Our computer is programmed to paint tumor volumes a bright fluorescent green—somewhere between a bright spring green and the foreboding yellow of a fire truck. It's done on purpose so that arteries in red or veins in blue will show up well against the background of the tumor. With one finger manipulating the mouse, I can turn a tumor around like a planet in orbit. I could look from the bottom, then spin it up and look from its "north pole," then move along its entire equator. I must have put that image of Sy's tumor through a hundred revolutions.

There were three things I absolutely hated about this tumor. First, the computer had been unable to draw a sharp border around it. There appeared to be a phosphorescent green haze, which meant the tumor was melting into the brain in such a way that the edges were not easily distinguished from normal, functioning brain. In no uncertain terms this was a tumor with microscopic tentacles into the surrounding brain.

Second, there was a nest of blood vessels just off the south pole—a knot made up of two smaller red threads intertwined with a larger, looping blue vessel. I could see that this tangle of vessels provided a significant blood supply to the tumor. More ominously, the green spheroid of the tumor swallowed up the red and blue lines. They disappeared into the belly of the tumor's mass, and there was no way to know where the vessels went. Off the lateral (outside) edge of the tumor was a single red line. Was it a second arterial feeder? Or was it one of the arteries from the bottom pole that had made its way up through the middle? If it was the latter, then it came out of the tumor and supplied normal, functioning brain as well.

The worst thing about this tumor was that it had chosen to grow in Sy Sonnenberg, its host. As I sank into bed around midnight, my last conscious thought was for him. How did Sy feel knowing that I would be sawing into his head in the morning? He knew, as I did, that there were no guarantees in neurosurgery.

Before any big surgery case, I have a ritual. I wake up early. It's almost always still dark whatever the time of year. I turn on the shower, steaming hot. I climb in and let the water wash over me for a few minutes. I wash my hair, my body, my face, and last, my hands. Then I remain under the shower and visualize the whole surgery in my head. It's as if I'm already in the OR. I imagine my eyes roaming over the operating table. I check to make sure all the right instruments are properly laid out. I see myself at the operating microscope and check all the lights on the power panel to make sure everything is working.

I visualize my OR team there, bending over computer screens. Then I see myself, always scrubbed in. I watch myself do the operation: from the first skin incision to the last closing suture. The operation seems to roll like a movie behind my closed eyes as I stand there in the shower. I'm walking myself through the whole operation. In my mind's eye, it's taking place in real time. Everything feels like it's happening at the same speed it would if I were actually in the operating room. But usually, when I look at the clock next to the shower, I've visualized the entire procedure in five minutes, no matter how long, or how complex the operation.

This morning ritual is my equivalent of a pilot's preflight checkout. I've discovered that the "inner eye" in my right brain can see potential problems that my analytic left brain can't identify. I envision the entire surgical procedure with the end result clearly in mind. I've rarely had an instance when the mental visualization led me astray. In the beginning, I had a hard time listening to my inner voice and trusting it, letting it guide me. But this visualization process has always worked. I get a pre-existing image of the surgery. I tap into it and it teaches me.

Over the years, I have had to unlearn a great deal of what I was taught as a resident. I was trained to believe that compulsive focus and a constant anxiety about the details is what would keep you out of trouble. As I grew older, I began to appreciate just how much luck has a role to play. When a surgical procedure goes well, it's not just our hands that pull it off. It's the patient, the anesthesiologist, the surgical team, and then a healthy component of divine intervention. There's a surgical adage that goes, "Better lucky than smart." This morning ritual of mine in the shower is my way of trying to get in touch with the invisible part of surgery, the part that you access through intuition, through the guts rather than through the cortex. You can get in touch with the divine powers. They can only be heard when a person silences his or her own mind. In the shower, I can turn myself off and listen. And ask for good luck.

In Sy's case, the shower ritual had been troubling. I wasn't concentrating well. The water was too hot, then too cold, falling too hard, then in my eyes. I couldn't settle myself down. Finally, I could visualize the tumor. It kept "bumping" into me. I would be working at the appropriate distance and focal length under the surgical microscope when it would suddenly jump out and seem to knock me back. It happened every time I got near that knot of vessels below the south pole of the tumor.

I imagined getting ready to tease the vessels apart. The blue vessel, the vein, tore. I could see blood coming from its wall. Not torrential bleeding, just oozing enough that I had to stop dissecting and turn my attention to it. I needed to reposition the operating microscope to look more closely at the vein in the bottom of the field of view. I coagulated it and moved the scope back to where I was working. In another moment, the vein started oozing again. I moved the scope again. I applied a small titanium clip to clamp the opening. The oozing stopped.

I turned the scope back to the tumor's main mass. But now the tumor was growing, turning a dusky, angry color. It rose up like leavened bread and pushed up toward me. I could see it was becoming engorged with blood. I moved quickly to resect the tumor. I finally got the ball of solid tumor out. And that's when I saw the single artery that was left behind bleeding. It squirted little red spurts at the edge of the resection.

As I went into surgery, I didn't understand what the vision in the shower was telling me. True, I was worried about the tumor's blood supply and how to best dissect the tumor volume. But I chalked the troubling vision up to a bad case of nerves—mostly the fact that it was Sy on the table and not a stranger.

Halfway into the operation, the true cause of my discomfort made itself clear. The vision had been meant to show me that the blood supply to the tumor was massive and that interrupting it would cause the tumor to swell. In resecting, I would have to sacrifice several vessels. But a critical one, the little arteriole that had waved at me like a flag in my shower ritual, now presented a horrifying reality. It not only supplied blood to the tumor but to an important area of the brain that was devoted to speech. I didn't have a choice. I had to sacrifice the small artery along with the tumor wall. I knew that as I coagulated it shut I might be sealing Sy's fate. I wondered if he would ever be able to say another word. If not, it would be my doing.

There's no loneliness like the solitary shadow that comes into a surgeon's heart when he or she suddenly realizes an irreversible error has been committed. That's one of the ironies of brain surgery. It's some of the most elegant and technically challenging surgery one can undertake. But that beauty carries with it a terrible price. You can make a mistake, hurt someone profoundly—where they live and think—and not be able to go back and undo your error. It's not like a piece of bowel, where you can cut a little more and stitch it back. The brain simply has no genetic capacity to regrow itself the way a muscle or a blood vessel does. One mistake and it's all over. It's the grace and curse of neurosurgery.

So when you make that irreversible mistake, it comes over you in the operating room like a sickening wave of darkness. No one else notices. Only you know that something awful has occurred beneath your fingers. The team keeps going about its business. The anesthesiologist's machines keep beeping unperturbed. The scrub tech keeps handing you instruments. On the outside you, the surgeon, just keep operating. On the inside, a frail human being is screaming to leave this place, get out of surgery. Just run! But you finish the case. That's the hardest part. You know something monstrous has happened. But you've got to finish the surgery, and then wake the patient up to determine if the damage was done. Sometimes you get lucky. You made the blunder but nothing happened to the patient. Then you feel great. Almost light-headed. But other times, you can't dodge the bullet.

It took almost two hours from when we removed the tumor to when we finished reconstructing the skull and closing all the layers of muscle and skin. The entire time, I had the feeling I was creating an elaborate sarcophagus out of living tissue. In the total darkness of the skull, deep in the brain, lay Sy's speech area in deathly repose. It had resisted the onslaught of the glioma. It had survived the tumor parasitizing its arterial blood supply. Over half the brain's normal blood was being siphoned off by the malignant tumor. But my hand had done it in. The speech functions had died where I'd sacrificed that last blood vessel.

I wheeled Sy back to the recovery area. He was still intubated. The soft elastic hose in his windpipe would remain until the anesthetic wore off enough for him to breathe easily on his own. Everyone knew Sy couldn't talk with an endotracheal tube down his throat. There was no way to move air across the larynx. But I knew a darker secret: he might not be able to talk even when the tube was removed. If Sy awoke mute, there was absolutely no hope that he could ever regain speech. I felt sure I'd dashed that hope during surgery.

I went out to Joanne in the waiting area. It was unbearable seeing the expectation in her eyes. She rushed forward, throwing her arms around me. I hugged her and whispered that the surgery was all over. I couldn't manage more. I said I would see her in thirty minutes in the intensive care unit.

In my office I stayed busy, dictating the operative report for Sy's surgery, which ran more than five single-spaced pages. I relived each excruciating moment, giving every detail about the large vein and the dangling arteriole. I felt like I was making a confession into the dictation machine.

It was time for me to go up and reexamine Sy. I put on a crisp, starched white coat and marched down the hallway toward the ICU entryway. As the automatic door swooshed open, I could see Joanne. She had her head in her hands, sobbing. A nurse was at her shoulder with a box of tissues. I watched Joanne kiss Sy's forehead and then his hand. As I approached them, I motioned for the clipboard and started looking over the vital signs. It was a way of diffusing the emotional tension.

Sy recognized me and extended his hand. I grasped it.

"Are you okay?" I asked. He smiled and nodded yes.

I didn't wait any longer. "What's your name?"

He looked like he would answer. Not a sound came out. His smile faded. He tried again, but nothing. There an odd look crossed his face— almost surprise but not quite. The room was absolutely quiet.

Then his expression changed and darkened. I saw the knowledge of his aphasia sinking in. Sy realized he couldn't talk.

I went on, holding out a pen. "What's this called?"

Silence.

"Is it a pen?" I asked.

He nodded.

"Is it a flashlight?"

He shook his head no.

I held up my wristwatch. "What's this called?"

Joanne had stopped sobbing, focusing intently on Sy's responses.

I dangled the watch in front of him. "Come on, Sy, what's this thing called?"

No answer.

My insides were churning, but I proceeded with the "examination." I jotted something on a notepad and held it in front of him.

Suddenly Sy smiled. I had written, "Stick out your tongue" on the paper. So he did—like a cocky kid.

Sy's response confirmed my suspicions. He could process and under- stand speech perfectly, but he couldn't utter a single word. Like a radio set that receives a signal perfectly but can't transmit sound. I had per- manently smashed the outgoing part of Sy's radio set.

I had to look away. I was afraid I was going to fall apart in front of everyone. I pretended to study something on his chart. My inner state was stark and miserable. I had failed Sy. My skills had failed us both. I was responsible for silencing one of the finest voices in neurology.

Neither Sy nor Joanne ever accused me of anything. They never even asked me what had happened. Once, Joanne mentioned that we had all known where the tumor was and that we always knew there was a risk. That was as close as we ever came to talking about it.

I suppose I could rationalize that I'm not responsible for the patient's anatomy. But it was my hand. There's a Latin axiom in medicine that states *Nihil nocere*. It means simply "Do no harm." I broke this most basic holy tenet. It didn't matter what anyone said or thought. I couldn't forgive myself.

I saw Sy and Joanne regularly as he proceeded through radiation treatment and then chemotherapy. The process pretty much followed what Donald had undergone. The drill for treating GBMs is pretty standard, and Sy knew better than anyone else how poor the prognosis was.

He stepped down as director of the Alzheimer's Research Center, and a national search for a new director started. He had just finished a $35 million fundraising drive, and construction on a new wing was moving along swiftly. He'd stroll along the site, almost daily, nodding and smiling. Joanne had developed almost telepathic skills and now seemed to be able to speak on Sy's behalf on almost any topic.

My agony persisted in silence. Like Sy's. Months later, when the tumor reappeared, none of us even mentioned surgery. Joanne remarked once that it was now a "mute" point.

As the new research wing neared completion, I suggested to the dean that it be named after Sy. They decided to have a gala event, while he was still alive. I had mixed feelings, of course. For me, it would be a painful blend of public humiliation and Sy's well-deserved recognition for decades of extraordinary scientific contribution.

I saw Sy and Joanne in the clinic about three days before the dedication and asked them how they were feeling about the coming ceremony. Joanne explained, as she now did out of habit, that Sy was excited and pleased everyone was making such a fuss about him. She also confided to me she had written a short speech and would read it on Sy's behalf.

As I sat there, listening to Joanne try to speak for Sy, I remembered an old, forgotten theory about brain function. It had been developed by a brilliant neurologist named Norm Mueller. He came to mind because Sy had been one of Mueller's own residents. Mueller's theory holds that certain types of speech function are locally specialized within specific locations in the brain. There's a transmitter region, usually located in the left, lower frontal lobe, called Broca's area. That's what had been irreversibly damaged in Sy's tumor resection. The theory also held that other areas, some of whose true locale and functions were still only hinted at, handled other unique functions (e.g., there's one area specifically for pronouns, one for prepositions, one for names).

One of Mueller's keen observations was that there were cases recorded in the medical literature about people who could not speak but could sing. Mueller was struck by the fact that the human central nervous system did not process musical sounds the same way it did the auditory patterns of speech. He had found and described several patients with strokes involving the left hemisphere who were aphasic like Sy. They couldn't utter a word. But...they could still sing!

I had so thoroughly given up any hope of Sy's ever being able to speak, so busy wallowing in my own recriminations that I never even thought of it. The Mueller theory held that musical ability would not be affected by damage localized to the inferior left frontal lobe. I wondered, could it be? Could Sy still sing? Suddenly, I found myself interrupting Joanne, who was talking about the dedication ceremony. I started blabbing about Dr. Mueller and then blurted out, "Joanne! Hold on just a minute."

I turned to Sy. "Sing 'Happy Birthday' for me, will ya? Come on, Sy. Sing!"

He stared at me in utter disbelief. Then he did it: he began to sing.

It was beautiful—as if he'd sung it a thousand times. To me, his voice suddenly seemed entirely magical. Joanne was just as startled and moved by the sound. She hadn't heard a word from her husband in months. He sang "Happy Birthday" again and again with a huge smile on his face.

We tried out half a dozen songs, like "Row, Row, Row Your Boat" and "Mary Had a Little Lamb." We had ourselves a little choral festival.

I looked at Sy. "Norm Mueller was a genius!" He smiled and sang a line from Gilbert and Sullivan in tribute to Dr. Mueller: "He polished up the handle so care-ful-ly, that now he is the ruler of the Queen's Na-vy!"

And so a strategy was born. Joanne took the little speech she had written on Sy's behalf and put it to music—to the tune of "Pop Goes the Weasel." It went like this:

> I'm really honored to be with you here
> To celebrate the new wing.
> I think it's so great that you named it for me
> Wow! That's amazing!

They practiced it day and night.

At the dedication, Sy went on for four stanzas. It was a wonderful, wacky, and moving performance. Of course, everyone had heard that Sy couldn't utter a word, so you can imagine the thunderous applause and the ovation when he finished singing his speech. I was in the back of the crowd, but I witnessed the magic, the power of it. I knew I had seen a miracle of neurophysiology and anatomical localization. It moved through all of us gathered there.

Sy lived for another eight months and sang out every single one. He would carefully practice each song with Joanne, sometimes working on them for days. Eventually he had different songs worked out for greeting, for thanking people, or for comforting fellow cancer victims. He actually became kind of a composer. As Wayne Dyer, the psychologist and writer admonishes us, you don't want to die with "the song in your heart still unsung." Sy didn't. To me, it seemed that a miraculous chorus was manifest.

I believe miracles do happen—incessantly. Like the Brownian motion of atoms, miracles are the backdrop of everyday existence. Miracles are the glue holding the cosmos together. We need only a pinch of hope and then the miracles appear. Hope waits for each of us to acknowledge it. I learned that from Donald and Sy. Next to love, hope is God's most potent manifestation.

Thirteen

For the Love of God

ome doctors secretly resent patients who not only experience profound religious transformations but also insist on introducing that faith into every aspect of their lives, including their maladies. It may be because many physicians equate religious beliefs with superstition and mystical symbolism. The truth is that I pity the physician who cannot envision medical science as an integral part of God's creation. I worry about a doctor who cannot see healing as an extension of God's love. Religious faith does not threaten scientific integrity. New medical discoveries need not be seen as nibbling away at God's preeminence and mystery. To the contrary, each new secret of medical science is nothing more than one more revelation of God's loving and majestic power.

Whenever I have a patient who can unabashedly affirm his or her faith in God, I heave a secret sigh of relief. I also feel a tinge of envy. The relief is because I know I have a foundation of authenticity on which to relate to that patient. I can feel comfortable making my concerns and doubts known to that patient. I feel freer as that person's physician to pray with him or her for a good outcome. The envy comes because, at times, I am not yet in possession of such unshakable faith. And I am afraid to exhibit it courageously at all times. That was why I envied Mrs. Hilts.

I met Louisiana Desirée Hilts in the pediatric neurosurgery clinic.

She looked ill to me, but I was struck by the energy and brightness in her blue eyes. In her arms was a child with poorly treated hydrocephalus— an abnormally large head caused by the continuous expansion of the ventricles without proper outlet. These children used to receive little medical attention. Fortunately, in the last three decades it has become a largely treatable condition, and only a very small percentage of babies fail to respond to today's surgical therapy.

In an adult, unchecked ventricular expansion would lead to death within a day or so (as it had in Donald's case). Neonatal hydrocephalics, however, are born with a soft skull made up of cartilaginous plates. As the ventricles push outward, the skull simply yields to the pressure and pushes upward and outward. Ultimately the head may reach several times normal size.

The child's name was Beau. Beau's enormous, baggy head was so heavy it had become a virtual anchor, pinning him down, preventing him from even looking around with his head. He displayed a classic clinical sign known as "setting sun sign," where the eyes looking downward in their sockets resemble the sun setting on the horizon. It is caused by the direct effect of increasing pressure on areas of the brain that control eye movements. His head was boggy. During examination, I felt the incomplete bony plates. It was also clear that the child's neurological development was severely delayed. Some intellectual impairment can be reversed with shunting—but much of it is permanent, as more than 60 percent of the central nervous system's development occurs in utero and in the first year of life.

I was absorbed in examining little Beau and had the tips of the stethoscope in my ears when Mrs. Hilts asked me a question. I could only hear a vague mumble. "What, ma'am?" I asked. I took the stethoscope out of one ear so I could hear better.

"Dr. Hamilton, I asked you if you had heard of Stonewall Jackson." An odd question. I nodded, a little annoyed that I was being interrupted in my physical examination.

"Yes, I do, ma'am. He was a famous general in the Confederate

Army, I believe. A great cavalryman, my grandfather told me. And he should know. He was a cavalry officer himself," I said.

"Oh, my! Did your grandfather fight in the War of Independence against the North?" She had a lovely, heavy Southern accent.

"No, ma'am. He fought for the Emperor and the Kaiser in the First World War. Had two horses shot out from underneath him."

"Oh, my," Mrs. Hilt gasped. "The Kaiser. Gracious! The Huns. Still, having your horses killed…that must have been terrible. No matter who you fight for."

"Yes, ma'am. I'm sure it was. He loved those horses dearly."

"Well, I can just imagine," she said.

"Yes, ma'am. You were mentioning Stonewall Jackson?"

"Well, I thought if you knew of Stonewall Jackson's fame, then you might want to know the general was little Beau's great-great-grandfather."

I looked down at the boy. He looked to me like nothing more than a "pumpkin head"—the unkind term we used privately to refer to these hapless children. "Interesting fact, ma'am," I murmured politely.

A few minutes of verbal interaction with Beau revealed the extent of his developmental delay. He couldn't utter a single word, at an age when most children can put together four- to six-word sentences and already have a sense of syntax. The circumference of his head was more than three standard deviations above the norm—quite literally off the growth chart. And because his head had weighed him down, he had failed to develop the truncal musculature and leg strength required for any mobility—even crawling. Everything had compounded itself in this little guy until he had become almost a caricature.

Creating a shunt from Beau's massively dilated cerebral ventricles into his abdomen would offer a conduit for the blocked cerebrospinal fluid. The trick with a pumpkin head is to be patient in the drainage procedure. To let the fluid out slowly over several days or even a week.

Because the hydrocephalic head is quite literally a big bag of skin with only a few flaps of bone down at the bottom, it can easily be overdrained, causing it to collapse, often tearing blood vessels in the process. In Beau's case, I planned a series of shunt adjustments, using a modern shunt that would allow me to reprogram the shutoff pressure of the valve, located behind the ear, by using an external magnet to reset the amount of drainage.

I planned to start Beau's valve with a fairly high pressure, so fluid would start running out of the shunt at a pretty good rate but not so fast that his head could deflate. In this slow process, Beau's head would shrink gradually and the bones would begin to adjust. I figured it could take as much as a year to bring his ventricular pressures down into normal range. Such an arrangement would let his brain respond slowly to the changes in cerebrospinal fluid and allow for the development of the other organs and systems in his body to catch up gradually.

The original shunt operation went very well. I used a ventriculoscope to look around inside his brain. I could see the cortical mantle of brain tissue, already badly thinned by the increasing pressure since conception. We nursed him postoperatively in the pediatric ICU. Within a day or two he brightened visibly. He began to eat better, almost as if his muscles had awakened from their slumber. He started making a few sounds—it seemed that his verbal behavior might pick up.

Over the next few months, Beau thrived. But Mrs. Hilts did not look well. One night, while finishing my evening rounds, I saw her sitting in a rocking chair, holding Beau. I was coming around because I wanted to adjust the pressure setting a bit in his programmable valve. Mrs. Hilts was ashen in color and nodding off despite her best efforts.

"Mrs. Hilts? May I pull up a chair for a moment?"

"Why, yes, of course, Dr. Hamilton."

"Thank you, ma'am." I settled myself on a stool. "Beau seems to be doing quite well, doesn't he? I think he is beginning to make progress."

"Do you think he will be of normal intelligence someday, doctor?"

"Well, that's hard to say. Many of these children end up being developmentally delayed for life. Just with the months and months of unrelenting hydrocephalus, some will normalize better than others."

"Would it be beyond reasonable hope that Beau could ever get close to what we might call normal? You know what I mean? Earn a wage, keep a checkbook, marry, have a family?"

I was recollecting how abnormally thin Beau's cortical mantle had appeared when I had just looked at it with the ventriculoscope.

"Mrs. Hilts, I don't really know, but I suspect not."

"I understand perfectly well, doctor. I just want to get a fair assessment of the terrain that lies ahead for my Beauregard. As his great-great-grandfather said, 'The understanding of terrain is what sets the stage for victory.'"

"Yes, ma'am. I think it's probable that Beau will need his family by his side to help him through life," I said.

"Precisely what has been weighing on my heart, doctor." She held a hand as delicate as dry parchment, fluttering momentarily over her chest. I could see her eyes filling with tears, which only served to make them more commanding. "I am dyin' of ovarian cancer, sir. This dear boy is my grandson, my flesh and blood. He was left in my care by his mother, who preferred drugs, alcohol, and fornication to attending to her responsibilities for her own child. She was completely unfit to be this child's mother and remains so till this day, I'm afraid. I am sorry to say this, as she is my own flesh and blood, but the truth is the truth. So, sir, Beauregard is my responsibility and mine alone. When you speak of a family by his side, I am that family, sir."

"I see, ma'am."

"I doubt if you can, Dr. Hamilton. For I can hardly see how I shall take care of this child while I am preparing to die. How can you have any realistic view of our dilemma? When I die, to whom shall the care of Beau fall?"

"I don't know," I answered automatically.

"I will not let Beau become a ward of the state. No, sir, I must pray and seek the Lord's guidance, for we are all His children and it is He who guides all of our footsteps. As Joseph said to the sons of Israel:

'God will surely visit you, and ye shall carry up my bones away hence with you.' So shall He come to our aid!"

With that, she cradled Beau tightly in her arms. Laying her head down, as if to shield him, she began to pray quite loudly and unashamedly. I bowed my own head.

"Lord, hear my prayer," she began. "I hold here in my arms your dearest son Beauregard. Lord, I do not fill your ears with complaints and protests. No, Lord, I ask only that you look down upon me and my tiny grandson and bestow upon us your wisdom and patience so that here, and in the future, Thy will may be done as it pertains to Beau and me. Lord, I realize that we are only passing time here on this Earth till we are able to rejoin you, our Heavenly Father, in Paradise. I ask for nothing but your guidance and love. Amen."

She opened her eyes and looked at me expectantly.

"Er...amen," I said.

With that, I took my leave. The next day I went over to the Cancer Center to talk with our expert in ovarian cancer, Steve Michelsen.

What he shared with me was grim: Mrs. Hilts had presented about a month earlier with what appeared to be intermittent bowel obstruction. Originally it was thought that she had diverticulitis. Exploratory surgery revealed, however, that it was advanced ovarian cancer, with hundreds of metastatic tumors coating her bowels, liver, and other abdominal organs. After they removed the primary tumor from her ovaries, there was little else they could offer. Michelsen told me flat out that Mrs. Hilts had only about ninety days left to live. I asked him if he had told her that. He hadn't. He had merely suggested that she might want to get her affairs in order.

Too often, physicians fail to be direct with their patients because they are not sure how to manage the delicate balance between dashing a patient's hope and retaining a patient's trust. I suggested that Dr. Michelsen and I sit down and discuss the situation candidly with Mrs. Hilts. I knew that her faith in God was very strong. Two days later, I went to meet them in a conference room at the Cancer Center. I had no idea just how powerful Mrs. Hilts's faith would truly prove to be.

Mrs. Hilts was already waiting. Her grandson was there, propped up preposterously in a little red wagon that came from the Pediatrics floor. His head lay on a large pillow. A hospital volunteer—a girl, actually—sat with him. His eyes seemed to flicker on her face without focus or recognition. Periodically she would insert into his mouth a pacifier that was pinned to his shirt. He would start up a round of furiously noisy sucking sounds until the pacifier slipped out, then start moaning till it was properly repositioned.

Mrs. Hilts sat at the head of the giant, polished wooden table. Behind her was a large picture window with a striking view of downtown Tucson. The brightness from outside, surrounding her like a halo, made it look as if she could be "swallowed up" in light. Like an angel. She might have chosen her seat expressly with that in mind. She was a woman of great presence and determination, that much was already apparent. A social worker was also at the table, leafing through a thin file and making checkmarks on some papers.

Michelsen arrived late. He was talking loudly into a cellphone when he entered. "Yeah, yeah. That's precisely what I said! You can take it or leave it!" He snapped the cover of his phone closed with the finality of a bear trap springing shut. It was inappropriate to have ended a conversation on that note in front of us. It may have inadvertently set the tone for what happened next.

"Yes, well, Mrs. Hilts! Forgive me for being tardy. I was held up in clinic."

"Dr. Michelsen, you are, of course, forgiven. I do hope that was your bookie you were talking to and not your wife."

"Bookie? Oh, no, no. That was..."

I thought to myself: this ought to be good.

"Never mind. I apologize," he said.

"Yes, Dr. Michelsen, you already mentioned your apology," Mrs. Hilts said.

"Yes, well, I'm sorry. I suppose we should get down...down to business, then. I've already kept you waiting." He pulled up a chair across from me, next to the social worker. "We have met...we are meeting rather...at the request of Dr. Hamilton," Dr. Michelsen began, "so we can better assess your illness and the impact...the effect this might have on the youngster here."

"Beauregard," insisted Mrs. Hilts.

"Yes, of course. Forgive me again, Mrs. Hilts. Your grandson, Beauregard."

"Well, it would seem to be my turn to be forgiven, Dr. Michelsen, as I was under the impression we were gathered here to discuss my cancer. And there was to follow some discussion, I trust, of the prognosis, if I am not mistaken."

Michelsen was on the ropes.

"Well...Yes, you are correct. That is what we are here to discuss. I...Dr. Hamilton...felt that because you are Beauregard's caretaker..."

"I'm his grandmother."

"His grandmother, I apologize. Because you are his grandmother and his primary care provider..."

"I thought a primary care provider was a doctor in internal medicine," she said. She was a tough old bird.

"No, I don't mean primary care provider. I mean you are functioning as his parent..."

He stopped, fully expecting her corrective interruption. But it never came.

He decided to try again. "Because you are for all intents and purposes his parent...his guardian, as it were, I thought it would be appropriate to discuss prognosis."

"Fine, Dr. Michelsen. I concur. Please proceed then with discussing my prognosis."

"As you know, 'prognosis' has different meanings to different people."

"It has only one to me, Dr. Michelsen. Survival," Mrs. Hilts said flatly.

"Yes, of course. Survival is the ultimate...well, it's one of the important parameters of prognosis. In your case, you have...very advanced disease."

"Dr. Michelsen, I am well aware of that. Could you, in fact, give me your best estimate of how long you think I might survive?"

"Survival is, naturally, a kind of statistic." He paused. "A measure, if you will, of how long a whole population of patients with your disease have been studied. Then the data collected. A median survival, a standard which tells us the central tendency, is established. In your case, the median survival—that is the point on the data sheet where 50 percent of the patients are alive and 50 percent are dead—that point is well...less, well, it's usually less than...four months."

"Are you, sir, telling me that I have less than four months to live?"

"No, no, Mrs. Hilts. No. I'm saying that if you were in the table of this data..."

"Doctor, the only table of which I am a part is the one at which you and I are both currently seated."

Michelsen flushed red with embarrassment. "No, I know. I'm aware of that, Mrs. Hilts. It's just that it's hard...it's tough to really give anyone specifics, because everyone is different. Everyone's disease is different. Every person is different."

He seemed to give up, ending on a pleading note.

Suddenly Beau let out a huge burp and started spitting up a milky fluid. Mrs. Hilts pulled out her handkerchief and wiped his mouth clean. She plunked the pacifier back in Beau's mouth. Then she pulled herself up quite erect and stood in front of the panoramic window. The light behind her became blinding.

"Dr. Michelsen, I completely understand your dilemma. It is, indeed, a difficult one. I appreciate that."

You could almost hear Michelsen's relief.

"I do not pretend to know what the future holds, sir, and neither should you. None of us has that power. Only the Lord Himself does, would you agree, Dr. Michelsen?" she asked.

He nodded in agreement. I saw the young volunteer next to Beau's red wagon also nod in agreement.

"So I would suggest a course of action, if I might, Dr. Michelsen."

"Of course. Anything... anything you want," he said.

"No, sir! It is not my wishes that must be met here. It is the Lord's. Do you understand that, Dr. Michelsen?"

"I'm not quite sure I do, Mrs. Hilts."

"Are you a churchgoing man, sir?"

"What?"

"Do you regularly attend church services, Dr. Michelsen? Do you or do you not? It's a simple question."

"I'm not a regular." He noted Mrs. Hilts's frown. "No, I do not attend... regularly, that is."

"In your line of work," Mrs. Hilts said, "that's a pity. I will read to you, sir, from the New Testament, Book of James, Chapter 1, Verse 5."

With that, Mrs. Hilts reached deep into her handbag and pulled out a small, worn, leather-bound Bible, put on reading glasses, and then stepped to the window. She turned sideways in the bright sunshine, now silhouetting her.

"If any of you lack wisdom," she read, "let him ask of God, that giveth to all men liberally and upbraideth not, and it shall be given him. But let him ask in faith, nothing wavering. For he that wavereth is like a wave of the sea driven with the wind and tossed. For let not that man think he shall receive any thing of the Lord. A double-minded man is unstable in all his ways."

She snapped the Bible shut, took off her glasses, and walked into the shadow of the corner. She was a consummate actress. At that moment, we were all in the palm of her hand.

"I am not a wave, Dr. Michelsen!" Mrs. Hilts asserted. "No, I am a rock! A rock made so by my absolute and unshakable faith in the Lord! I am not double-minded! I am single-minded in my purpose! I am totally focused on my allegiance to my God. Let His will be done!" She paused and looked over her audience. None of us dared to move a muscle. Like a preacher secure in the pulpit, she was on a roll.

"So while I am quite aware that my condition, stemming from this ovarian cancer, is—as Dr. Michelsen tried so eloquently to point out a moment ago—precarious, and represents a statistical long shot at being overcome, I do not bet against the Lord! No, sir! So I would not bet against me either! Since I am the Lord's foot soldier, I think that I shall stand quite well in His holy estimation. He looks with great benevolence upon those who are willing to pick up His shield and sword. I subjugate myself and this dear child to His infinite love, mercy, and, most of all, His will. So let us undertake all manner of therapy secure in the belief that God's will, and God's will alone, will be done here. Is that understood?"

Michelsen just nodded.

"The Lord has given me this child for a reason. I cannot imagine that He would place this dear, retarded child in my care if He did not intend for me to be here to take care of him. So I have prayed to the Lord to give me the strength and resolve to endure and survive all of your chemotherapy, Dr. Michelsen. I believe that the Lord will assist me utterly to succeed. In that, I have more faith than you can imagine."

With that, she turned, took the handle of Beau's little red wagon, and departed.

Michelsen put his head in his hands. "What in the name of hell just happened?" he asked, looking over at me.

"I think she just appointed God to be her primary care provider," I muttered. The social services worker smiled shyly.

"Well, I warned her. I want a note put in her record documenting our discussion here today," Dr. Michelsen said to the social worker taking notes.

The discussion was, in fact, memorialized succinctly by the social worker. It read:

Dr. Michelsen told Mrs. Hilts of the grave prognosis of stage IV metastatic ovarian cancer and gave her an estimated survival of four months.

Mrs. Hilts acknowledged the Doctor's comments and asserted that she had no intention of dying because she believed that the Lord had other plans for her.

Mrs. Hilts proved to be correct. The Lord had a completely different idea. Beau made an astonishing recovery in his intellectual abilities and eventually went on to trade school, where he learned how to build beautiful, ornate birdhouses. One of them is currently in the meditation garden of the Cancer Center not thirty-five yards from the conference room where Mrs. Hilts read to us from the Bible that day. Beau also got married. His grandmother was at his wedding.

Less than three years after Dr. Michelsen declared her unlikely to live more than four months, Mrs. Hilts attended the doctor's funeral. He had died from his own hand, from an overdose of sleeping pills and alcohol. She sat holding the same little Bible and laid a rose from her own garden on his coffin.

Last year, at the ripe old age of eighty-eight, Mrs. Hilts spoke the following words to a cancer survivor group:

"You need to be a realist to believe in miracles, because one can only see the real truth with the heart and not with the eyes."

Amen.

Fourteen

The Surgeon Who Became a Murderer

Confusion now hath made his masterpiece!
Most sacrilegious murder hath broke ope
The Lord's anointed temple, and stole thence
The life o' the building!
Shakespeare, *Macbeth* II, iii

have always maintained that any reasonably well-intentioned medical student can become a surgeon. But only good character ensures a mediocre surgeon can become a great one in the passage of time. Surgeons, in that regard, are a lot like wines. One must attend to the details of nourishment, such as soil, terrain, rainfall, and nutrient supply. Then there is the matter of the vines themselves, which must have the correct pedigree, the right heritage. Then there's the matter of luck. Luck always plays a part. Weather, ripening, the cool wind rolling in just when it should, making the harvest. Then comes the science of fermentation, proper aging, and the great wooden casks in which the wine will rest and sleep, waiting. Then comes the opportunity to taste it. It's only then that you will be able to tell if you have that rare vintage of which all have been dreaming. Anything less and you've just got expensive, ruined grape juice.

Never forget that all-important, essential, large, heaping spoonful of luck. What one is to become is largely predetermined by forces beyond our control. We don't choose who our parents will be. We can't dictate when and if one of them will leave us or die. We can't shape the values that are evidenced by the grown-ups around us. Yet all of these may have profound effects on our character, and in the end, that character may dictate our destiny. So I do not hold that we make our own destiny. We ride it. Wherever it'll lead us, to wherever we are supposed to end up.

By the time awareness arose within me about how and why my values were shaped, it was too late for me to exert that much effect on the outcome. What if my stepfather hadn't taken me to Sagamore Hill? What about the draft and Dr. Denin, the veterinarian? There may have been one or two exceptional moments, I suppose, where extraordinary willful acts on my part might have helped to steer me in one direction or another. I am afraid, however, that even that sensibility of discipline and self-determination draws its inspiration from an earlier stage in life for which we are hardly able to assume responsibility.

It is an intriguing exercise to go behind closed doors and see, as the chairman of the Department of Surgery, how the top candidates for entry in the residency program are selected. There is a great deal of competition surrounding surgical residency. There are fewer than a thousand residency slots open each year in the United States. The competition is intense, because so much of the struggle focuses on the top 25 percent of the programs. In addition, many of those slots are what we refer to as "preliminary" positions, as opposed to the categorical ones. Everyone wants the categorical ones. "Prelim" positions in a residency program guarantee only a year or two of training, focusing on the first year of internship, and sometimes include a second year of junior residency. There is an explicit understanding that no one selected for a prelim position will be there for more than one or two years. These slots are far less attractive, and therefore the rivalry involved in the selection of medical students for these positions is reduced.

Categorical positions, on the other hand, are reserved for the very best individuals in each year's crop of graduates, and these positions are for the entire five-year span of the residency program. Categorical candidates are chosen with the implicit understanding that they'll finish their training as qualified surgeons as long as they are physically and emotionally able to do so. The rivalry for categorical positions at the best programs becomes white-hot in its intensity.

Usually there has been a very extensive but mechanical assessment of applications in order to make a determination of which candidates will be chosen to interview. This first cut is almost entirely statistical. A complicated mathematical formula adds up the candidate's scores from national medical examinations, as well as a point scale for honors, as well as a scoring system for the quality of the letters of recommendation on the candidate's behalf. A computer digests all this mathematical scoring and then formulaically spits out a list of candidates who are invited to be interviewed, starting with the highest-scoring and working down the list, with the cutoff being usually at about the top 25 percent.

Once the applicants actually arrive for interviews, the evaluations of the different interviewers are also scored, and ultimately, between the first set of equations and the second, candidates are placed in a rank order from most desirable to least. But before the list is finally submitted to the agency responsible for the National Residency Match, there is one final faculty meeting. Sometimes we refer to this jokingly as the "human meeting."

The human meeting occurs forty-eight hours before the final match list has to go in, and it's an opportunity for the faculty to see the list and add its own human insight into the equation. Here, a faculty member might try to appeal on behalf of a candidate he or she knows well. Conversely, if a surgeon has a terrible experience with one particular candidate, and yet that applicant scored very high on the proposed list, this is where a faculty member can come forward and condemn a candidate, resulting in placement at a much lower position in the list. On occasion, there can even be factions emerging, where some faculty are lobbying hard on behalf of one candidate while other groups stand up to forcefully oppose it. At times, the human meeting can be very much a political process, with clear-cut splinter groups and parties. Deals are cut. Votes are taken. Compromises created.

The decisions made there have enormous repercussions for the applicants. A medical student in the top six is essentially guaranteed his or her choice of surgical positions, as there are six categorical slots at our institution each year. Of course, some of the candidates we rank in the top ten or twelve slots may choose to go to better or more prestigious programs. Obviously, if we are keen on getting someone in our program, other programs will want this person too, by and large. That is why the National Match is so critical: because each residency applicant also submits a list in which he or she rank-orders the programs, with number one being the program into which the graduate would most like to be accepted. A giant computer then matches the student's choices against the teaching institutions. It's a giant residency lottery.

A great program prides itself on "getting its top choices." So, for example, a great surgical dynasty like Duke (or Harvard) might never have to go below its sixth-ranked applicant to fill all six of its residency positions. That means the top candidates also chose that institution as the most desirable. A less prestigious program might have to dip down on the list to the thirtieth or fiftieth position to fill its six categorical slots. The worst programs don't match; that is to say, all the candidates they wanted in their program were snatched up by better programs. That scenario is a flat-out disaster. All the data about how resident applicants were ultimately matched up with each program is published annually. Furthermore, the results show how far down its "wish list" a program had to go before it filled all its slots. So a program that received its top five candidates is given kudos for being a very desirable, prestigious program, while another that had to dip as low as its seventy-fifth candidate—or worse, did not fill all of its slots—earns a reputation as a bottom feeder, a program on the skids. So the data published on the selection of candidates has a great influence on the national reputation of a program. It is the subject of intense rivalry among academic institutions.

Still, occasionally a categorical resident, even one good enough, smart enough, and lucky enough to have gotten a categorical position, has to leave. Something can happen. A resident develops cancer. Or someone decides to take a position closer to home. Once in a while, sadly, a resident throws himself out a window. Then a categorical position opens up unexpectedly. With none of the intense competition and scrutiny of the traditional match. It is almost up for grabs and will fall to the person who spots it when it's first announced over the Internet. Such a position may even be snapped up internally by someone in a prelim who might have proven herself or himself good enough for consideration. A great deal of luck is involved in many residency decisions, and the unexpected categorical opening really takes on the flavor of a Las Vegas high-stakes poker game.

Mike Dent got into our program after one of our original categoricals had to drop out of the program. At first glance, Mike had the look of a winner. Like he might prove to be a great vintage. His had not been the typical straight path from premed to a research lab to med school. Mike had come up the hard way. His parents had been dirt-poor ranchers along the Mexican border in Douglas, Arizona. They'd seen drought. Border smugglers stealing through the landscape at night, taking a calf or two. And they'd seen golf resorts spring up out of the desert where folks came in and spent more money installing a wet bar by the pool than Mike's family had ever earned in three generations of hardscrabble cattle ranching.

Nonetheless, Mike had grown up well enough. He had entered law enforcement. As a Border Patrol agent, he'd distinguished himself by showing compassion and courage on the job. He had found and saved dozens of illegals making their way along the treacherous desert border crossing. Despite ruinous influences that seep across the U.S./Mexican border—where the staggering riches of the United States are juxtaposed against the deprivation and poverty of Mexico—Mike saw his role as one he was privileged to fill. He'd even met a beautiful señorita to whom he gave his heart, and he eventually obtained her hand in marriage.

Together they hatched a plan in which they could better serve humanity together: Isabella would go to nursing school and Mike would study hard at night to get into medical school. He planned to become a surgeon. Isabella would be his trusted ally in health care, and together they would return to Douglas and start a clinic, open to patients from both sides of "the line." It was a nice dream for the two of them and for the people they ultimately would serve.

Both worked hard at this dream. Isabella became an ICU nurse. Mike made his way through medical school and was ultimately accepted into a categorical position that suddenly opened in my surgical residency. They managed to have two beautiful children along the way. Isabella landed a great job heading up a surgical nursing team at the University Medical Center—a position usually reserved for nurses with more than twenty years' seniority.

For the first two years, Mike was the epitome of the "blue-collar" surgeon. That is just what you might expect: he took serious care of his patients, but always seemed to be able to poke fun at himself and take everything in stride. He appeared to get along with people from every stratum of society, from the well-heeled to the down-and-out. He had a gift for connecting with people.

Over the course of the third year—the "hump" year—where surgical residents turn from "grunts" into technically proficient surgeons, Mike and Isabella grew apart. That's not uncommon. Many marriages fall apart around the middle of surgical residency. Mike was no longer the heroic officer in the desert. He now carried thirty or forty-plus pounds on what had once been a lean, muscular frame. This is often referred to in the business as the "surgical gut." He looked more like a used-car salesman than the tanned, rugged specimen he had once been.

Was it his fault? No. He had used those magnificent years Jung called "the years of the athlete and the warrior" burning the midnight oil. His youth had been spent on his studies and the rigors of residency. Stress had been building up between the couple as Mike progressed through the program. The single-mindedness he needed to survive and finish his training dimmed all other needs. He saw the kids less and less often. He would fix that all later, once he had survived surgical residency, and started up his own practice. That's what we all tell ourselves.

Somewhere in the course of events, Mike came to see me. He admitted that when he came home, he'd swill down a beer or two, eat in a hurry, and collapse into sleep. Sometimes he needed a sleeping pill. His libido had left him. He found himself screaming more at home and enjoying his wife and family less. He simply came to me to request that we change his on-call rotation to give him rest and some sorely needed time with his family. I met with my senior administrative staff and we all agreed to comply with Mike's request. We recognized the severe strain under which both Mike and Isabella were living. We arranged for couples' counseling. We tried to do what was right.

Not everyone agreed with my decision. Changing the residency rotation schedule in the middle of the year is hardly something that goes unnoticed. I remember an angry confrontation in my office when several of Mike's fellow residents came to see me. They believed it was blatantly unfair of me to modify Mike's schedule. Why couldn't they all make the same request? Shouldn't their needs also be considered? Besides, some asserted, in a surgical residency program, all residents were expected to prove their resolve, show their mettle through thick and thin. This was a rite of passage. In their eyes, I had also violated an unwritten code of honor. What they were saying was true. But there were compelling reasons to believe that Mike and Isabella might be near the breaking point in their marriage.

Whose side to take? I couldn't reveal to the angry residents the problems Mike had confided in me. In their eyes, I had made an unfair and arbitrary decision. From my perspective, Mike was in deeper trouble than they were and he needed rescuing right now. I told the angry delegation of residents that they would simply have to trust me. I had the best interests of the program at heart. I knew what I was doing. They didn't really believe me, though.

Mike and Isabella went to counseling. Mike seemed to rally. I didn't see much of Isabella. Word was their marriage was done.

One Friday afternoon, my secretary called me to tell me there was a detective at her desk. A detective? My mind went right to my own family. At the same moment, my pager went off—the last three digits were 911. That meant the ER, and I had to be there stat! All I could think was that one of my kids had been in an accident and was already in the ER. Since the detective was right there, I ignored the pages. He introduced himself. He immediately assured me the matter had nothing to do with my family. He asked me if I knew a "Michael Eliot Dent."

I told him Mike was one of my residents. "What's up? Is he okay?" I asked.

"Well, sir, I have bad news. We found his body today...this afternoon," he answered.

"His body?"

"We have reason to believe that Dr. Dent shot his wife several times and then took his own life."

"Oh, God," I moaned.

The door to my office flew open. It was two of the residents who had been part of the group that had met with me a few months earlier. Their faces were pale.

"It's Isabella and Mike! They're coming! They're coming to the hospital!"

This was close to overload. We not only had to deal with the emotional tragedy, but now both victims were coming through our own doors. I asked the detective calmly where Mike's kids were. Both were in emotional shock having come home from school to find their parents shot. I told the detective to contact Mike's parents in Douglas and to help them find their way to Tucson as fast as possible so they could help with their grandchildren.

On automatic pilot, I put on my white coat under the wide-eyed stares of my two residents. The next two hours were a blur of horror.

Isabella, who still had a pulse when the officers found her, arrived first. Mike had shot her five times, twice in the chest. A third bullet had gone through her jaw and exited behind her eye. We slashed through her chest wall to insert tubes. So much blood. We went through all the motions. But it was futile. We quit trying finally, half of us crying, all of us covered in blood. We looked like jackals around a carcass.

Mike arrived with much less fanfare in the trauma bay next to Isabella's. They lay there side by side, stripped of their clothing. Maybe they hadn't been that close to each other naked in a long time, I thought to myself.

Mike had done a thorough job on himself. There was no way he could have been saved. He had put the gun squarely in the back of his mouth and pulled the trigger. We pronounced them both dead and turned the scene over to the police.

In Mike's pocket, the police found a court order informing him that Isabella was seeking a divorce. He had received the notice at work. Attorneys can be thorough when serving papers like that. Mike had read the letter on lunch break. He had calmly handed his beeper over to the senior resident on his team, along with a complete list of his patients and their medical issues and anticipated pending tests. Mike told his resident that he was joining his wife for a late lunch. They had, he said, some things to work out. Then Mike went home and shot her and himself.

With Mike and Isabella now officially dead, all of the surgeons had nothing left to do. We just stood around helplessly as the body bags came out and toe tags were applied. Too many forensic photos had to be taken. It was heartbreaking.

I asked the surgical faculty to take call for the residents and we sent as many residents as we could home to be with their families. But what would they be able to say? To their wives? Their sweethearts? That one of our own had gone crazy and shot his wife, the mother of their children, and then himself? I busied myself with the minutiae of informing the dean. I also contacted a psychiatrist and two psychological counselors and told them to ready themselves for convening all the residents early the next morning. The press was already swarming all over the entrance of the ER. Microphones and TV cameras collided with us around every corner. We briefed our own public relations team and sent them to draw the press away. We needed to be alone.

At seven the next morning, we met in the amphitheater with all the residents. I told them the facts as we knew them. Mike's and Isabella's families had decided to have a joint funeral service for both in the same church in Douglas. Both families asked for the coffins to be laid side by side next to each other.

For all of us in the amphitheater, the grieving and counseling process was just beginning. Gradually, emotions began pouring out into the meeting hall—predominantly, at first, rage at Mike. One resident after another expressed anger that Mike had not just committed suicide. Why did he murder the mother of his children? Leave them orphaned? How could a surgeon, who had sworn to save lives, take another's life? Over and over, expressions of shock, then shame, emerged from the assembled residents.

As the counselors skillfully encouraged people to get in touch with their feelings and to share the sorrow of having both Mike and Isabella in the ER, they also gave advice on grieving the deaths. There was resistance on the part of several to feel sadness or pity for Mike.

"Why should I feel sorry for that bastard?" a senior yelled out from his seat in the auditorium. A lot of heads nodded in assent.

"Yeah," said another. "He's a murderer. And look at what he's done to the reputation of the program!" The story was making national headlines, and my office was being inundated with e-mails and faxes indicating that applicants were requesting withdrawal from consideration for the coming year in our residency program.

One of the counselors asked us all aloud, "What do you think might have made Mike do such a thing?"

There was a long silence in the hall. An intern suggested that maybe Mike was "emotionally disturbed."

The counselor asked what Mike had been like as a resident and colleague. Answers slowly began to come forward that he was a good guy. He worked hard. He stayed late to take care of his patients. He always lent a hand. He was a team player. He was compassionate. He seemed to have a special place in his heart for the Mexican illegals that came into the ER. They had moved nearly 180 degrees from their earlier position.

The counselor summed it up: "Sounds like Mike was a pretty great guy, doesn't it?"

A few heads nodded.

"It sounds as if Mike was once an exemplary surgical resident, doesn't it? Like he brought great dedication to his work? And great credit to the program?"

More heads nodded. You could hear one or two sniffles.

The counselor went on. "It sounds as if Mike just snapped. Right?"

The room grew silent.

"I guess it worries each of us that we could snap like Mike did, that we could all work so hard to be good and yet be capable of something like that," the counselor said.

The whole amphitheater was numb. The counselor had gotten to the heart of the matter. It could happen to any one of us. That was why we were all in such turmoil. You didn't need to be malevolent. You didn't need to be evil. You could be a wonderful human being and still commit a horrible act.

As surgeons we must bear a peculiar burden. We try to hone ourselves into instruments of service. We must resolve to do no harm. But surgery requires a delicate administration of violence, real violence. It takes will and practice before a person can pick up a knife and cut open a fellow human being. It takes years of training until a person gets the right feel and knows just how much pressure to exert to compel the tissues to open. As surgeons, we all know in our guts that every surgery is only a hair's breadth away from murder. Of course, there is a great moral difference between an act that may result in death and one that is deliberate killing. Surgeons work within those terrible borders. By overcoming the necessary barriers to becoming proficient at surgery, we may also risk lowering the barriers to other kinds of violence. Maybe an occupational hazard of sorts.

Like every surgeon, Mike had to dwell occasionally on the razor's edge of madness. There are so many factors that can unbalance a surgeon. The unshakable operative confidence, driven by the high-octane fuel of the ego. The almost unbearable loneliness of putting one's technique against a patient's disease. The tension that comes from repeatedly playing with the lives of others. The sleep deprivation that gradually gnaws at one's self-restraint, eroding patience, and even, at times, forgiveness. And last, there is luck—the final factor in the breakdown. Bad luck in Mike's case. The impact of receiving divorce papers made him, on that day, at that moment, snap. Unbalanced, he tipped over into the abyss, swallowed up in darkness and despair.

As the chairman of Surgery, I did not think the surgical residency ever quite recovered its former status as a premier training program after Isabella's murder and Mike's suicide. That kind of thing stays with you and the story sticks. A decade later, when two surgeons chat about the merits of the various surgical training programs, the murder will come up. Long after all of the surgical faculty have retired and a couple of hundred residents have finished training and gone into practice, the murder will be there, reposing in the collective memory. When those of us who must remember finally pass away, then maybe the ghosts can depart. Until then, we are each haunted by whatever connection we had to Mike. There is a sense of communal guilt that a murderer moved among us, stood with us in our ranks, and we did not do enough to stop him. We train hard as surgeons because we believe each life is sacred. To take one by accident is a sin each surgeon must learn to live with. But to take a human life on purpose—that of another or one's own—goes beyond personal sin. Even in the depths of war, there is certain anonymity to how we inflict death upon an enemy. The bomb that falls kills at random. Without conscience. Without selective intent. But Mike selected two particular lives to be ended with malice and purpose and forethought. To the extent that my surgical program selected him and trained him—that it happened while I was in charge—makes me an accomplice in his crime.

Fifteen

Luck of the Draw

I hope good luck lies in odd numbers, either in nativity, chance, or death.
SHAKESPEARE,
The Merry Wives of Windsor, V, 1.2

uck, good fortune, fate—whatever one wishes to call it—is a slippery notion. It has an elusive quality, like quicksilver. It runs in strange directions. It defies reason. I've tried to show how mercurial a role it has played in my own life and in the lives of my patients. How can you embrace luck at the same time that you scoff at hope? Hope is essential to every surgeon. Hope is the flip side of luck.

I like a surgeon who carries a lucky rabbit's foot in his pocket. Or a four-leaf clover in his wallet. A surgeon without luck is as hapless as a sailor without wind.

Much of my neurosurgical practice is devoted to brain tumors. I've had the honor of taking care of hundreds of patients with astrocytomas, malignant brain cancers. Very few survive for more than a couple of years. As I mentioned, the odds for long-term survival can be a thousand to one. To be "cured" one needs to be lucky indeed—it's a real long shot.

Thank goodness every neurosurgeon who deals with astrocytomas has at least some survivors. Without this handful of the lucky few, this glimmer of hope, it would be difficult to keep going. As surgeons, of course, we must often resign ourselves to our patients' unfortunate outcomes. But it's human nature to want to step up to the plate and "hit one out of the ballpark." You need to "connect occasionally to keep swinging," as one of my surgical mentors told me. Without hope, it's hard to operate.

I've had two "home-run" astrocytoma patients. They—and I—have been very lucky. One's named Rusty and the other Paul. They're very different from each other. Rusty is an alcoholic, chain-smoking, ne'er-do-well. Thus far, he's learned to attach himself to women and convince them to love him, to take care of him. And of course, he also has a brain tumor. Needless to say, he's charming, and could play that brain tumor tune well—like a concert violinist.

Paul, in contrast, was a busy engineering student. I met him shortly after he suffered his first seizure that led to the discovery of a malignant astrocytoma. I resected it a week later. The severity of subsequent radiation and chemotherapy forced him to suspend his studies for an entire semester. The following year, however, he returned to his master's degree with a vengeance. He managed to push through chemotherapy. On the final scans at the completion of treatment, there was no visible trace of a tumor. He got married and started working on his Ph.D. Soon he and his wife were hoping to settle down in Berkeley, California, and start a family as soon as Paul finished his dissertation.

Rusty, in the meantime, would come into clinic with his latest girlfriend. Usually he reeked of booze, and sometimes he was downright obnoxious. When he was drunk, he had a habit of hanging off my shoulder as if he were my best buddy. Or he'd come swaggering down the hall, yelling, "Hey, doc! How ya doin'? Hey, let me introduce you two. This here's Rose, my girlfriend. Come on over here, sweetie, and give Daddy a smooch, will ya? The doc don't mind, do ya, doc?"

"Well," I'd say, "I do sort of mind. It's nice to meet you, Rose. Rusty, come sit down. Behave yourself. Let's get on with the exam." I'd scold him.

"Sure, sure, Doc," he'd answer. "But let me get my smooch first, eh, Rose? I'll behave myself a lot better if I get my smooch, doc."

Other times, he could be disarmingly innocent. I was once looking over one of his routine CT scans. Up to this point, Rusty's tumor had been confined to the left frontal lobe. On this newest scan, it seemed to have progressed across some of the white matter bundles (called the corpus callosum). It had begun to spread to the right hemisphere. In neurosurgery, we call this phenomenon "bihemispheric spread." It's considered a very bad sign. I took out my pen and traced the ominous path that the tumor had taken so Rusty could visualize it better.

"Wow!" he said. "That doesn't look good, does it?"

"No," I said, "not a bit. It's definitely a sign the tumor is progressing."

Rusty was about two years out from the time of his original diagnosis. He had lived with three different girlfriends during that interval, but had recently moved in with his mother, who lived on a meager Social Security pension. She'd driven him forty miles to help him keep his appointment that day.

"Ma, this doesn't look good, eh?" Rusty asked, looking over at his mom.

She had tears in her eyes. "Don't you worry, Rusty," she said. "It'll be all right."

"Yeah, that's what I figure, Ma. But let's ask the doc. How long do I have?" he asked me directly.

I can never give a clear answer to that question, because there isn't one. And as I mentioned earlier, a surgeon has to be careful not to extinguish the patient's hope. I wanted to be candid, but the fact was I'd never had a patient survive more than six weeks after an astrocytoma had spread to the opposite hemisphere.

"Well, doc?" Rusty said. "How long? A few weeks...months?"

I was stalling, pondering exactly what to say.

"What? Six months? Or maybe a year?" he prodded.

"No. I doubt a year, Rusty. Possibly six months or so. You know, a good three to six months, I suppose...maybe."

Rusty's face turned somber, and he directed his gaze downward to hide it from his mom. She was holding back a sob, dabbing her eyes intently. Then Rusty had a renewed burst of energy. He looked up with a big smile and touched the cigarette he always kept tucked behind his left ear.

"Well," he said, "if it's only a few months, then let's make the best of it. Right, Ma? And if it's not gonna be all that long, maybe I should think about getting into a hospice program or something, you know? Get out of Mom's way. What do you think, doc?"

"I guess that depends on what the two of you want," I said. I explained I could get him set up in a program right near where they lived so he could be close to his mom and she could visit him easily.

"Well, that'll be good," said Rusty. "That'll give Ma a little more peace and quiet. Won't it, Ma?"

His mother showed some relief at hearing Rusty suggest that he move out and go into a hospice program. I don't think she really wanted to feel that way, but having him home was surely not easy. He'd already been arrested in her '73 Buick for two DUIs and had lost his license.

"You don't have to go to hospice," his mother said. "You can stay with me. You should stay with me. We'll be okay, you'll see."

"No, Ma. I really want to do this. It's okay, isn't it, doc? I mean, for me to head over to hospice?"

Of course it was okay. My office made the arrangements. The hospice medical director helped Rusty get settled. The hospice had a shuttle van that could take him around wherever he needed. He could even visit his mom regularly, have a few beers out of her fridge, and then return to the hospice building.

During this same time period, Paul's scans remained pristinely clean of any recurrent tumor. He'd been able to finish up a very challenging doctoral dissertation. Our whole clinic staff attended his graduation. We threw a small party for him in our staff lunchroom before he headed to Berkeley with his wife. There were five candles on the "birthday" cake one of the nurses had baked—one for each year he'd survived from his initial diagnosis. He was my first five-year survivor. When one looked at his scans, there was every reason to believe that Paul was cured of his disease. That was something all of us in the clinic wanted to celebrate, as much for ourselves as for Paul.

At the party, one of our nurses brought a third-year med student over to meet Paul while I was handing out slices of cake. She announced, "This is Paul. He's a doctor of engineering and a five-year survivor of brain cancer." The nurse beamed up at Paul, just as proud as if she were his own mother. The medical student obviously knew already how rare it was for anyone to see a five-year survivor of an astrocytoma. We could see the disbelief on her face. Paul chuckled at her surprise.

"It's true," he said. "I'm five years out... and still counting. Have a slice of cake."

Rusty, meanwhile, had been taken twice to the Sierra Vista Medical Center with seizures. We suspected they were brought on by his alcohol abuse, but with an underlying tumor like his, we had to rescan him every time. Each scan looked exactly like its predecessor; no bleeding, no further growth. Just this big, ugly tumor straddling both hemispheres. I'd look over each scan and reassure myself that Rusty was no worse. The ER physician would load him up with a couple of doses of anticonvulsant to forestall further seizures. Rusty would then go back to hospice.

I saw Rusty routinely and reviewed his scans on each visit.

"How's it look, doc? Any better?" he'd ask.

"Nope. It's no better. No worse. Looks exactly the same. There's been no change."

"Well, that's good news at least. Hear that, Ma? No growth. No change. We're holding our own!" he'd crow.

Rusty could be so upbeat. His mom seemed to cheer up. Hell, Rusty could even cheer me up.

Two months after his last visit, the hospice director in Sierra Vista called me up on the phone. I figured Rusty had probably had another seizure.

"Listen, Dr. Hamilton, I've got to discuss how we're going to deal with Rusty," she said.

"I don't know what you mean," I said.

"It's just that... well, Rusty has been here for over six months and he seems to be doing just fine. He seems okay. We usually don't have patients, or don't let patients, stay in hospice for over six months. That's sort of our maximum, if you know what I mean."

"They usually die by then," I said.

"Well, yes. I'm afraid so. Hospice is essentially designed around the terminally ill. And frankly, Rusty seems no closer to dying than when he started here. I don't mean it like it's a bad thing. It's not a criticism or anything like that."

"No. I know what you mean. You're right in a lot of ways," I said. "His scans sure suggest he should've been long gone by now. That's why we sent him to you in the first place."

"I know. But we've got to use the beds for patients who really are dying. We're going to have to send him back to his mom. I'm sorry, that's just the way we have to function here."

"I understand."

"Do you want me to tell Rusty and his mom, or are you going to handle it?" she said.

"I should be the one to talk it over with him," I said. "I can just tell him, 'I've got great news for you: you flunked out of hospice.'"

I set up an appointment for Rusty and his mother to see me. When I walked in, I could see they must have been expecting bad news. I quickly took out the CT scans. Absolutely rock stable. No change whatever, I reassured him. I explained the dilemma that had arisen about Rusty's staying in hospice.

Rusty, the eternal optimist, took the news about leaving hospice gleefully. "Wow, that's great! I get out of hospice, Ma! That means I'm doin' better, eh, doc?"

I nodded. "Yep. I guess that's right."

"So what's goin' on with my tumor?" he asked.

"I can't really explain it, Rusty. But for some reason, your cancer has stopped in its tracks. It looks like it just quit growing. At least for now, for the time being."

"Doc, that's great news!" He jumped up and embraced me and

then grabbed his bewildered mother and dragged her into the midst of our hug.

"Doc, that's just the greatest news I could ever get. Man, am I gonna celebrate," he said with a wink in my direction. I knew exactly what he meant, but I couldn't blame him. I'd never had a patient get expelled from hospice. It was something to celebrate.

Over the next three to four years, Rusty and Paul both would regularly get CT scans. Paul would dutifully send me his follow-up films from California. I would look at them and discuss the results with him and his wife by phone. Rusty, on the other hand, would return every three months with his mom. I grew accustomed to Rusty's tumor scans remaining unchanged. Paul's scans stayed completely clean.

I began to feel comfortable relaxing the follow-up schedule. We would repeat scans every six months instead of every three. Eventually, I moved the schedule out to once a year. When one of their scans would come up for review at our Brain Tumor Teaching Conference, everyone would gasp in amazement. Paul's was what we'd always imagined a brain cancer cure should look like—entirely normal. Rusty's scan also blew everyone away—for different reasons. His tumor defied all logic. It seemed to have just gone to sleep.

Like an afterthought, Rusty married his steady girlfriend, Lucy, after a year together. The marriage was rocky at best and lasted only two years, and then Rusty started coming back to see me with his mom as his companion again. Paul had two children in the interim and had taken a faculty position at Cal Tech, where he was promoted to associate professor with tenure.

After thirteen years, in 2003, when I saw Rusty again in clinic, his scan hadn't changed one bit. I treated him with a nicotine patch so he could finally try to quit smoking. He figured if he'd been alive for this long, it was probably time for him to take his health more seriously. He still drank excessively, but he settled down with his mom and became a pretty good cook for the two of them. These days he always gets shown around to med students and residents like a VIP when he comes in. He takes off his hat and shows his craniotomy scars proudly.

"Yep," he says parting his hair, "I flunked hospice and I'm still alive to prove it. Ain't I, doc?"

In 2003, Paul reached almost fourteen years out from diagnosis. He and his wife had just finished building a little place in the hills about two hours' drive from their home near Cal Tech. That same year, Paul had a seizure. I got a repeat scan in California just to be sure and had it sent out to me for review. I looked it over in disbelief. There was a new spot. It had never been there before. A new tumor to kill. Paul had to come back and undergo a course of focused radiation, aimed at killing the tumor. Although this original spot disappeared from his subsequent scans—and we have to assume the tumor with it—the recurrence changed Paul profoundly. Where before he believed he had achieved a miraculous cure—so had I—now he was haunted by the notion that his tumor was stalking him, lurking among the shadows of his MRIs. Biding its time. And symbolically, now, he was looking over his shoulder. Something he'd never done before. And I looked with him, peering with the aid of the latest technology—like MR spectroscopy and PET scans, searching for telltale signs. But with each follow-up scan we no longer celebrated. Now it was just a sigh of relief.

I have learned that luck, good or bad, can spell the difference between surviving and perishing. It can be the power behind a successful surgery or a frightening complication. And luck seems, at times, to be the farthest beyond our control just when it can exert the most influence over whether we live or die. We have to just accept it: patient and physician. I have not mastered how to rejoice when we can enjoy good luck but not feel embittered when luck turns bad. So many of my patients impressed me (especially some whose stories I've shared with you). Patients like Rocky, Candy, Taylor, Donald, and Sy did not rail against fate. Each of them left this life after acquiring a sense of being at peace with the world when the moment to depart finally came. They had embraced their luck—good, bad, or indifferent. I still struggle to learn from their examples. To draw inspiration from the dignity and strength they lent to me just because I was fortunate enough to serve as their surgeon. But I still experience moments—years after they have passed away—when I cry for some of them. And for myself. So few home runs.

Sixteen

Soul Survivor

've been sharing some of my own "rounds" with you. Not because they're so special. Just the opposite. Many of the spiritual experiences I've written about are *not* unique. They're common, everyday events you'd find in every medical center. And although I can't vouch for those of other surgeons, the majority of these experiences get overlooked—dismissed.

Why? Why was it that when a spiritual experience happened on my watch, and when I saw it with own two eyes, I would always first tell myself it was a coincidence? My first reaction was to write the episodes off. They appeared to be distractions, luring me off course from the larger task of completing training as a surgeon. Later, however, these experiences became vital ingredients to my own perception of my life's work. Many of them begged the larger issues of spirituality, extrasensory capabilities, and supernatural forces.

When I search for what's remarkable in my career, I realize it hasn't been the surgeries I've performed. The spiritual connections seem the most memorable ones and the most worthy of sharing. Beyond technical feats in the operating room lies an opportunity to assess our own values, our own perception of our singular mortal existence, and deciphering whatever greater meaning it may hold.

No one warned me, during the various stages of my surgical career, that as I entered into the lives of patients, I would have to wrestle with my own life to discover my personal priorities. That my character would be tested and my integrity would be challenged. And that I would feel humbled and humiliated by my shortcomings. No one told me you couldn't undertake major surgery—as patient or doctor—without opening yourself up to spiritual realignment and, sometimes, outright transformation. I should have suspected it. But I've finally come far enough in my own development to know that every surgery offers me the opportunity to step farther into my own uncharted spiritual territory. Every patient steers me closer to my soul's purpose.

A recent case—the last patient we will visit together in this book—offered me a unique opportunity to evaluate what may lie beyond our mortal life. It occurred at an outside medical institution. The case was so unusual, so appealing in its summary facts, I felt compelled to travel up to Phoenix to talk directly with the health care personnel involved, as well as with the patient. I wanted access to all the records. I asked to see more than the usual materials in the medical chart—additional items beyond blood pressure, core body temperature readings, and EKG documents. I wanted to review the three hundred sheets of continuous brain wave recordings. I asked for both the video and audio tracks that had been taped during the surgical procedure. In addition, there were several videotaped interviews with the patient to be scrutinized. I felt like a detective, armed with a search warrant.

I was not the only one asking to see them. Other doctors, researchers, and experts on consciousness were making similar requests as word of the case spread through the local medical community. Few of us, as doctors, suspected we might encounter something altogether new or unique. The vast majority of us who investigated this case thought we would eventually find a mundane, rational explanation for what had happened. That once again, inevitably, the seemingly miraculous would be deflated. This was the reason we desperately needed to make sure the records—"the line of evidence," so to speak—did not get befouled until no one would later be able to decipher them. We feared that, because of inadequate or ambiguous documentation, we might not be able to give a logical explanation for this seemingly unusual case. We came with the purpose of explaining it away. What we stumbled on instead was a unique opportunity to evaluate the potential for consciousness beyond the physical, biological, and physiological borders of the human brain. In short, we would have to ask ourselves: Could the mind have an existence entirely independent of the central nervous system? For me, this case offered a once-in-a-lifetime chance.

The case involved a thirty-four-year-old woman who was under the care of Thomas Reed at the Barrow Neurological Institute. I had known Thomas for more than fifteen years and judged him to be among a handful of the most gifted neurovascular surgeons in the world. The woman worked at an architectural firm. While at her desk one day, she suddenly experienced twinkling lights all over the room. "They flashed like Christmas tree lights everywhere," as she had described it. "Right after that came a blinding headache. I felt like someone had driven a knife right into the center of my head. Then I must have fainted, because when I came to, my coworkers were all standing around me. I just grabbed my head with both hands. I felt like it was going to explode."

She had, in fact, suffered a relatively small but almost lethal intracerebral hemorrhage. The source of the bleed eventually was pinpointed to what is referred to as a "basilar tip aneurysm." Basilar aneurysms are nothing for the faint of heart. The vessels that branch out directly from the basilar artery feed most of the important areas of the brain stem, regions that account for breathing, swallowing, and even regulating the heart's rhythm. When something goes amiss with a basilar artery aneurysm, the patient almost invariably dies. But this woman hadn't, and that meant her basilar aneurysm would need to be repaired.

This particular aneurysm was challenging from a technical perspective. The swollen, ballooned portion of the aneurysm had actually engulfed and surrounded two important arteries that could simply not be injured or sacrificed. The aneurysm had swelled, like a rising loaf of bread, and would have to be teased off both blood vessels before it could be definitively repaired. But how to do this? Almost for certain, dissecting the aneurysm in this fashion would cause it to rupture—in which case, she was dead for sure. But what if there was no blood to spill out when it did rupture? What if there was no flow at all?

The surgical team decided to address the repair by cooling the patient's body temperature down low enough to put her into a state of suspended animation. To make her core temperature cold enough to stop her heart so all blood flow would cease—maybe for as long as twenty minutes. To accomplish this goal, the young woman's body would have to be slowly cooled on a heart-lung bypass machine, a device that oxygenates and then pumps the blood back into the patient's body. Eventually, as the body's temperature dropped below 90 degrees Fahrenheit, her heart would stop beating altogether. Once it stopped, the bypass machine would also be shut down. All blood flow to her body and brain would then cease entirely. At that point, all her brain wave activity on an EEG monitor would fall to zero. Then the aneurysm could be approached without being obscured by bleeding. It would be clipped under deep hypothermia. No more than twenty minutes could be allowed to complete this task. By then, if all went well, Dr. Reed would have the aneurysm successfully clipped so it would be completely excluded from the circulating blood flow. When the deadline was reached, the bypass machine would be turned back on. Her blood could then be slowly and progressively rewarmed. We hoped that as her body temperature returned closer to normal, the young woman's heart would resume beating. As blood began surging again through the brain, everyone hoped it would revive from its cold torpor and the production of normal brain wave activity would be restored. That, at least, was the plan.

The patient was, understandably, scared to death. Tom had given her odds that there might be as much as a 50 percent chance she would die on the table. Without surgical repair, as risky as it was, there was a 100 percent chance she would die. Sobbing, she signed the consent for what is, without doubt, one of the riskiest operations in all of surgery. Less than two dozen times had this kind of cardiac standstill been used for brain surgery. Mishaps, strokes, heart attacks had plagued many of these first attempts. In two cases, the patient's blood supply never returned to life.

It's an everyday occurrence in cardiac surgery to place patients in situations where they undergo a planned cardiac arrest—technically referred to as cardioplegia, because the heart stops contracting. In these scenarios, a heart-lung bypass machine replaces the heart's vital pumping function. This is done so the heart no longer has to contract and is not a "moving target" while the cardiac surgeon operates on it. But in the case of basilar artery aneurysm surgery, there is one crucial difference: all blood flow is allowed to completely cease for a period of time. Here, even the heart-lung bypass machine gets turned off. There is absolutely no blood flow in any blood vessel (including the arteries feeding the brain) until the basilar artery is repaired. Stopping the heart-lung bypass machine is never permitted to happen during cardiac surgery while the patient's heart isn't pumping. Unless, of course, the patient has died. Then it becomes the final act in an intraoperative death.

Under normal, physiological conditions the brain simply will not tolerate being deprived of its blood flow for more than two to four minutes. Longer than that and the brain dies. Instantly. Irrevocably. The period of time the brain can tolerate complete cessation of blood flow can be extended by cooling the brain down. The lower the brain's temperature, the less oxygen is required to keep individual neurons metabolically viable. There are some remarkable accounts of individuals—especially children (whose smaller bodies cool more quickly than adults)—who have survived without any discernible brain damage after being completely submerged in frigid waters for periods of up to forty minutes. Usually this happens after the individual has fallen through the ice on a body of water in the winter. While we understand the physiology, it still is no cakewalk to pull this stunt off in the operating room. A lot of luck is required. Like a successful rocket launch, it's spectacular when it comes off without a hitch. And a horrifying crash when it doesn't.

From a technical point of view, everything required for this daring surgical undertaking went well. Without a hitch. The patient's body cooled, the heart stopped as expected, and the brain waves disappeared. She was dead by every clinical criterion used in modern medicine. During her brief interval of seventeen minutes "as a corpse," while a titanium aneurysm clip was carefully put into its final position, forever sealing the aneurysm off, the surgeon and the OR team worked and exchanged few pleasantries. Most of the conversation centered on the operative and technical concerns at hand. Surgeon and assistant would mutter quietly as they gazed through the microscope, working on the delicate blood vessel. The anesthesiologist watched his instruments but had time to chat with the nurses while everyone waited for the aneurysm clip to be positioned and then closed, finally, quelling the danger of the aneurysm forever.

Most of the conversation was lighthearted. There's a video and audio track documenting the operation through the microscope. The audio portion is simply a recording of whatever ambient noise is picked up on a small boom microphone. Nothing fancy. A microphone like the kind one would pick up at Radio Shack. This audio track would eventually prove to be one of the most important pieces of evidence we would sift through.

As the operation began to wind down, several trivial conversations were picked up. One part related to a conversation between Tom Reed and the perfusionist, the technician who oversees the heart-lung bypass pump.

"We're going to need to start the pump back up in a minute or two. Everything ready to go?" Tom asked.

"Yeah, we'll be ready. We've got to blow first," the perfusionist answered. To "blow" is vernacular for firing up the pump and letting it circulate for a few seconds to ensure any bubbles in the system are cleared before reestablishing blood flow in the patient. While the pump was readied, there was a second important conversation picked up by the microphone. One of the nurses in the operating room, a certain Rita Hightower, announced she had just gotten engaged. A couple of the other nurses shrieked in excitement. Because Rita was scrubbed in, wearing surgical gloves, she wore no engagement ring.

But she said, "Oh, wait till you see it. It's a one-and-a-half-carat square-cut yellow diamond. And he proposed to me right there at Morton's. John got down on his knees and proposed. In fact, one of the waiters didn't see him and tripped and fell into the wine case. Nothing broken, but it was funny." A couple of oohs and ahhs. Someone in the background asked where the ring was from. "Johnston Fellows." This was one of the most exclusive shops in the Phoenix area. "John had it custom-made for me."

The pump was cleared. "Thar she blows, captain," came the answer.

"Okay, then. Let's pump this baby up, shall we?"

The bypass machine churned and red blood began to flow again through the patient's tissue. The patient's body was gently rewarmed. Her heart started beating again. A few minutes later a normal, healthy brain wave pattern reappeared on the EEG. The operation by Dr. Reed went flawlessly. But there was one matter that troubled everyone. That was why I felt compelled to go see things for myself.

As the patient awoke in the intensive care unit, she emerged gradually from the grogginess left by all the anesthetic agents. After several hours, her head cleared. She sat up to greet Dr. Reed and his team of residents when they stopped in to see her in the evening.

"How did everything go today?" the patient asked.

"Textbook-perfect," Tom said with a smile. He quickly examined her. All of it was recorded on the video camera in her room.

"Well, I thought I remembered hearing something 'blow' during the case," she said. "Did the aneurysm blow?"

"No." Tom must have gone sheet-white. I could not see, as his back was toward the stationary camera in the corner.

"I thought someone said, 'Thar she blows.' Like in *Moby-Dick*."

"Yes, well that…what you might have heard…was the tech telling me all the air bubbles were blown clear out of the lines. That's all."

"Oh. I'm glad. I was just remembering what a disaster you said it would be if the aneurysm leaked or ruptured."

"No. Everything went fine with the aneurysm." Tom leaned in closer to the young patient. "Is there anything else you recall?"

"Yes, a ring. A one-and-a-half-carat yellow diamond from Johnston Fellows. Oh…and Morton's restaurant where someone fell into a wine case."

Tom just kept staring at her. "You remember all that?"

"Yes. Why? What does it mean?"

"Well, those were just conversations we had in the operating room. Nothing special."

Tom left the room and immediately paged the anesthesiologist.

"She remembers what happened in the OR!"

"No. No way!" answered the anesthesiologist. "No, it's impossible."

"Well, you come here and ask her what she remembers!" The anesthesiologist came up a minute later and charged into the room and made her repeat word for word everything she could remember. He began to scratch his head and muttered, "How the hell could this happen?"

What shook everyone up who watched the video between Tom and his young patient was we all knew that this woman's brain had been dead—without discernible electrical activity whatsoever. This meant that no brain cells were active, working, firing, or emitting electrical signals. Yet somehow the patient managed to recall the conversation in the operating room while her EEG was flat. In other words, while she was, for all intents and purposes, clinically dead—with no ability for her brain to function—she somehow managed to make or "encode" specific memories of that conversation in the OR. And this was no hazy recollection. The patient was reproducing practically word for word what had been said. Right down to the jewelry store and the waiter stumbling. No, she clearly recalled what had been said. There was no doubt about that.

From everything we currently know about how the brain works, it would be utterly impossible, from a biochemical, metabolic, and physiologic point of view, for this woman's brain to create a memory. To do so would require neurons to be activated and then be capable of encoding incoming electrical signals. This electrical activity would cause them to convert the voltage signals across the cell's surface membrane into specific changes in the transcription of messenger RNA—or mRNA—in each neuron. These changes in mRNA produce precise molecular changes, altering amino acid and peptide production within thousands of cells to make a lasting memory the brain can recall. In order to create a "Kodak moment of recollection," the brain must be very much alive and bristling with electrical activation, and intracellular metabolism must be "revved up" to the maximum of each cell's capacity.

Yet we also had here unequivocal, scientific evidence that not only was her brain *not* working, it specifically demonstrated the absence of *all* cortical electrical activity when these conversations actually took place. So where could these brand-new memories have been created? Where had these memories gone? And where could such a place exist? Certainly, wherever it was, it would have to be beyond the confines of her own brain and mind as we currently understand them. But wherever these memories existed while her brain ceased to function, how could they be accessed later from such a location? And how could such memories survive intact "out in the ether," a place accessible to her brain for later storage only after it revived and awoke? One thing was clear: Explanation or not, she had stored and recalled accurate memories of what had happened.

We would have to come up with some new explanations. One theory held that her brain—and the conscious mind it produced—went somewhere else, beyond its own physical and physiological confines. Out into the cosmos. The notion that conscious awareness—something generated by and of each brain—could have a life (so to speak) independent from the brain itself is a baffling idea. To us, as physicians, at least. Maybe not to Tibetan Buddhism or other faiths that believe in reincarnation.

Another notion, just as radical as the first, was advanced by a group of physics researchers. Their idea was that the memories of the conversation in the OR could survive intact as discrete quanta of energy. This is similar in concept to rays of light from stars, lying far beyond our own galaxy, reaching us here on Earth. The light we perceive tonight was actually sent millions of years ago in the past. In fact, the star whose light reaches our retinas today may have actually extinguished itself long ago. The quanta of light we perceive exist independently from the star. In a similar fashion, once the quanta—the packets of "memory energy"—came into existence, they might become independent of any brain's ability to remember them. Later, supposedly, these quanta could somehow be available to reenter the brain. So just as the light waves we see today in our telescopes came into being millions of years ago in a distant star, memories could persist independently in the cosmos until the individual's brain was ready and able to "experience" them.

Imagine, for a moment, the implications of the notion that quanta of conscious energy could exist independently in the Universe, able to enter from anywhere, at any time. Maybe they might even go into someone else's brain that was not even present, where the memories were never intended to reside. And if intended, by whom or what? Could such intention be exerted by an unconscious or "brain-dead" patient? All of this also was leading us into unfamiliar territory, where theoretical physics merged with the realms of consciousness. Where our notions of being alive and aware now intermingled with quantum mechanics and the stars themselves.

No matter how we sought to explain it, this woman's experience seemed to indicate that the mind, the essential repository of consciousness, could somehow be induced to separate from the very brain that created it. That it could live without neuronal support of any kind. Maybe her "deathlike state" was a prerequisite condition.

This was why so many doctors and researchers now flocked to Scottsdale to see the patient and pore over the records and data. The personnel in the OR were scrupulously and independently interviewed to ensure that no one individual's recall would become contaminated by hearing the recollections of someone else. The patient was also interviewed and videotaped separately. All OR personnel (besides Tom and the anesthesiologist) were asked not to see the patient. The patient became the equivalent of a valuable archaeological find. We wanted to leave the site undisturbed.

We began our inquiry with a vague, almost smug, scientific curiosity. We felt confident we'd find a plausible explanation that would make this seeming mystery disappear. We began by eliminating the obvious explanations. For example, we needed to be absolutely sure that no one—including the patient herself—could have heard about the conversation in the operating room secondhand or thirdhand from someone else. As the more rational explanations faded away one by one, we began to wonder if maybe we had encountered something unique. Wondrous even. Could we be looking at the neurophysiologic equivalent of the Holy Grail? Were we holding solid, convincing evidence that consciousness could exist wholly separate from the brain? Perhaps even generated outside the central nervous system rather than being its by-product? None of us—scientists or physicians—could ever have imagined that one day we night be close to a vindication of individual awareness beyond the brain. In fact, this particular patient's consciousness seemed to thrive despite substantial evidence that her brain was concurrently dead, incapable of generating a single electrical impulse.

To put this into an everyday context, it would be equivalent to stumbling upon a lightbulb (consciousness) that could stay illuminated without any electricity (the brain). All along we had believed the lightbulb could only generate light when electrical current flowed though it to make the filament glow brilliantly. Given our present findings in Tom's patient, we were faced with a radical new paradigm: bulbs don't need electricity at all to glow. But then we must ask ourselves: If bulbs don't need the flow of current, then how do they work?

We met again with the patient. Her name was Sarah Gideon, a petite brunette with a closely bobbed haircut reminiscent of Dorothy Hamill. She had two children, both boys, ages five and eight. With both kids now in school, Sarah had just started working as a receptionist for a leading architectural firm in Phoenix. Her favorite pastime was quilting—something she often did with her mother and sister. She was Catholic and had attended a religiously oriented school run by the Carmelite Sisters. She went to church services but "not as much as I should," she added. "But I go for, like, the holy days. Around Easter, Palm Sunday, Christmas, or Christmas Eve." She told me she prayed every night before going to bed but rarely read the Bible outside of church.

"Have you ever had an out-of-body experience before?" I asked.

"Is that what happened to me?"

"No, no. I don't know. None of us really do," I stammered.

"Is there something wrong with me? With my brain?"

"No. Not at all. It's just when you came up to the ICU, you recalled so much of the conversation from the operating room. That's, well, that's never happened. It's not supposed to…under circumstances like…the conditions of your surgery. Do you have any recollection of being in the operating room? Of looking down from above? Maybe of seeing yourself on the operating table?" I asked.

"No," she answered, almost brusquely. "I'm sorry. I don't remember anything. Just what I heard."

"Do you remember hearing the voices? Hearing people speak?"

"Yes and no. I can tell if it's a woman's voice, for example. But I don't know what she looked like."

"What do you imagine," I asked, "say, about the woman you heard discussing her engagement? What do you think she might look like?"

Sally looked down at the nurse's call light button in her hand. A look of sadness came across her face. "I imagine," Sarah confessed, "she's blonde. About five foot six. Petite. Wearing a surgical mask and hat."

"What color eyes?"

"Blue." She concentrated on the call light. Like she might have to call for help.

"Does the hat on her head look like a large surgical hat? Pulled over her head like a shower cap?"

"Yes. I think so."

"Sarah...how do you know she's blonde? Which she is, by the way."

She closed her eyes. "Because I think there was a curl of blonde hair showing. Sticking out. Like it had fallen out. Onto her forehead."

As I quizzed her for further details, it was obvious she had an image of everyone in the operating room. There were so many little facets that she knew. For example, she was able to tell me exactly where the heart-lung bypass was located in the suite. Yet it had only been brought in after she was under general anesthesia for more than two hours. In other words, she could not have seen the machine before surgery began. Sarah also knew the pump technician had a beard. She told me the second scrub nurse was African-American and very tall. In fact, she was over six feet tall.

What emerged from the several conversations I had with Sarah over the next two days was that she was aware of the room, its occupants, and the conversations that took place within it. Her consciousness was present in the operating theater even though it was not supported in any way by her brain.

There was now a tantalizing context in which to understand much of what I had experienced in my own career. The dream of Tan-Beang that guided me so many years ago. Rocky's son coming back to him the night before his death. Thomas's father coming back from the grave to watch over his son and make sure that the gift of life returned to his boy. Harry's premonition and, later, his wife almost joining him. Alfred's death working its way physically into my back. And the unshakable Mrs. Hilts.

These past interactions seemed to link my own experience as a physician with supernatural forces exerted by others or manifested through others. Could we, I now wondered, be connected together beyond the abilities of our individual brains to sense and comprehend?

A great school of fish, made up of thousands of shimmering individuals, is capable of swerving instantly as a unit without the awareness or insight of each fish in the group. Could it be that, like the individual fish, I had mistakenly believed the journey I was undertaking was mine alone? Instead, perhaps, it was the journey of many, forged from myriad physical existences that were interwoven into a fabric of consciousness far beyond the reach of our senses or the grasp of our intellect. Perhaps we are like the gathering school of fish, steadfastly maintaining we are single individuals while our collective awareness moves us freely into unrecognizable depths. Maybe some fish look upward and see the sunlight filtering down and wonder, "What do these ripples I see above mean?" Do the ripples, like the supernatural eddies I experienced on the clinical surface of medicine, suggest there are other realms beyond the confines of our ocean, what we have accepted always as our one true reality? Can that particular fish see a ripple and imagine continents with jungles, mountains, polar ice caps, and deserts?

So what do we, in the field of medicine, do with unsettling disturbances, the supernatural ripples? Ignore them? Ban their discussion? Or do we declare them simply to be a puzzling mixture of science and spirit? Can we not, as doctors, allow ourselves to entertain the possibility that the supernatural, the divine, and the magical may all underlie our physical world? Would we not be the richer for just challenging our imaginations? Don't we owe it to those who come after us to at least raise the questions? Can we not admit we yearn to glimpse the mystery of the spirit? And we need to ask questions when we stumble across evidence that consciousness survives beyond the life of the brain.

I'm reminded of a carved angel that lies closest to the top of the spire of the Notre Dame cathedral in Paris. She is turning away from the cross just above her, and she shields her eyes with her arm and hand. It is rumored that the artist depicted her this way to indicate she has been struck blind after seeing the glory of God. So perhaps Sarah's experience and memories are as close as we can get—just a glimpse, but one that suddenly turns our world of scientific convention and constraints on its head. It may well be that we can survive and even expand into realms far beyond the physical restrictions we have learned to accept as inviolate over thousands of years of scientific observation and research. As

Blaise Pascal, the French mathematician and philosopher, wrote, "God could make it all obvious, but at a terrible price." So remembering the lesson of the brash angel, we must content ourselves with this oblique glimpse and trust that, for now, as much has been revealed as we can withstand, for our own good. We cannot grasp it. Or measure it. Or map it. But maybe it has to suffice for now.

I know if I have questions, so too will other doctors and patients who come after me. This is my turn to speak up. I am doing so because I feel that maybe, for the first time in my own life and career, I know what I'm supposed to do. I'm not looking for extrinsic guidance from my peers or the scientific literature. I am content to be just what I am: amazed and excited about the possibilities. I tell you this: Whatever solitude we feel on our journey through life is entirely of our own fabrication. We are the only judges who can sentence us to solitary confinement. We alone are empowered to make a conscious decision to envision and embrace our spirituality. Our susceptibility to feel connected to the supernatural is enhanced by experiencing the uncertainty of severe illness, the anxiety of major surgery, and the sheer fragility of life. But in these three lies the shimmering gateway.

Sarah was discharged a day after my last conversation with her. So much was left unsettled, unanswered. First, a heated dispute erupted between two physicians in the hospital cafeteria. One, a British anesthesiologist named Sir Newton Pitcairn, was a revered authority in the field of the application of quantum physics to the science of consciousness. Sir Newton felt there was no doubt that Sarah's case was a straightforward demonstration of consciousness being separate and independent from the brain's state of activity. This view was thoroughly rejected by a neurophysiologist from my own institution, the University of Arizona, who called into question "the degree of electrocerebral silence evidenced by the EEG record." In other words, he did not believe Sarah's brain had been totally asleep during the surgery.

To satisfy myself, I took a copy of the EEG and showed it to two more colleagues in Neurology who routinely read EEG printouts for a living. I told each one of them that this particular EEG was taken from a patient whom I was asked to declare "brain-dead." In short, this was someone whose brain was believed to be completely destroyed, and I wanted to be sure there was no evidence of brain wave activity. Both of them assured me that the EEG was unequivocal: the patient's brain was dead. A goner. So the case left us squabbling among ourselves, dividing into camps.

Sarah, however, left me with a far more disturbing question. I had asked her: Did this experience—of recollection of what had been said in the operating room—change in any way any of her presumptions about life? Or God?

"Yes," she said. "I have faith. I believe in God. I know that when I die, I will be with Him in Heaven. For all eternity. So the incident reminded me that I do believe."

"I believe in God too," I said.

"Yes, but you want me to reassure you that God is there. You want to know that I was somehow out there with Him. You're asking me all these questions because of your own doubts, your own fears."

"Maybe so. I just want to…"

"You just want to *know*! Not believe. Like I do. But know. For sure."

"I suppose," I said.

"Did it ever occur to you that the reason I may have experienced whatever I did—whatever you and your colleagues are running around trying to prove—might just be a reflection of my faith?"

"I'm not sure what you mean."

"I believe in God so I'm able to join Him. You don't—or you worry that maybe you don't—so you can't."

I just stared at Sarah, dumbfounded. She was absolutely right about my desire to know. About my doubts. I thanked her for her time. I embraced her. I had nothing left to ask her. Nothing left to say. I left. It was my turn to ponder, to try to answer the query. I never saw her again.

Six months later, a documentary special came out on one of the networks. It was entitled "Back from the Dead." It was sensationalistic, filled with jerky camera work, reenactments, and snippets from experts, including Sir Newton, silhouetted dramatically against a graveyard.

A year afterward, while on her way home from the architecture firm, a dump truck ran a red light and killed Sarah instantly. She died from massive head injuries. In her autopsy report, the Maricopa County medical examiner described the massive head injuries that Sarah had suffered. As she dissected the base of the brain away from the skull, a metallic gleam caught her eye. She peered under the edge of the temporal lobe and saw the titanium clip. Tom had taken such care to place it in position on the basilar aneurysm. It had required such effort, teamwork, and precision. And the circulatory arrest required to put the clip in position had raised such perplexing questions about Sarah's consciousness. The pathologist removed the brain and placed it in a bath of formalin, turning the brain over to better visualize the tiny little clip. She dictated into her microphone, "A titanium clip is found in good position, securely around the neck of an old basilar aneurysm. It is unrelated to the patient's cause of death and is mentioned in this case only as a finding that is incidental." To me, that clip was hardly incidental. Given the issues Sarah's case raised, perhaps, more like transcendental.

Decent Interval

When I began writing this collection, there was no way of foresee-ing that my own journey might take an unexpected turn. In many of my patients' stories, I've been trying to underscore a sense that life is full of "unexpectations"—unpredictable, destabilizing surprises. As someone said, "Do the gods exist? I don't know, but they sure act like they do!" So the gods played a joke on me. You'd think I would have expected something like this. But I didn't even see it coming. I was just coldcocked, knocked out in the first round.

In 2004, I had to undergo major reconstructive surgery on my lower spine. It had all added up: the earlier spine injury in Desert Storm, maybe a disk rupture after Alfred's death, and, finally, getting bucked off a horse. My luck had run out. My spine started aching during long surgical cases. Eventually I couldn't ignore it. My left leg became numb with every long surgery I did. Then my right leg started burning. Weak-ness settled in my left limb. I started to worry my legs might give out, buckle under me at just the wrong time, at a delicate moment during surgery. Ironically, I had always been aware a human body might fail during a surgical procedure—but not my own. Never had I reason to doubt my own ability to see an operation—every operation—through to its conclusion. But now I did.

MRI studies showed that I was at risk of becoming paralyzed in both lower extremities from compression of the cauda equina, the bottom part of the spinal cord. I had no choice: I had to become a patient. And I had to make up my mind quickly before the unthinkable happened. So I went under the knife. And I surrendered, knowing surgery can fail, no matter how hard we wish it to succeed. If surgery could end well—without risk—then it wouldn't be surgery as we know it. Without chance, luck, fate, it can't be surgery. They're all vital ingredients of the recipe.

My surgery was more complicated than planned. A projected two-hour case turned into ten hours of surgery. I lost nearly half my blood volume. The surgeon labored to reconstruct my spine with titanium and fuse it with dowels fashioned from my pelvis. He slaved over my spine as if his own life were at stake. Even now I feel sorry for him, imagining what he endured to finish the case—our case. Later, I discovered I would not make a complete recovery.

In my bed in the ICU, I began to discern a certain anxiety in my colleagues' eyes as they visited politely with me. I could see some veiled fear in their eyes. What have they seen or heard, I wondered, that they aren't telling me? Maybe a suspicion that I'll never be strong enough to perform surgery again. Maybe I was seeing that secret dread all surgeons share: giving up the scalpel. I've known surgeons who committed suicide rather than live without operating. So much time and energy have been sacrificed to finally become surgeons. Many of us can no longer see a life without it. Metaphorically speaking, we want to save our last heartbeat for the operating room, as unbelievable as it may sound.

That fear made me feel helpless. All surgeons fear an operation can go too far, to a point where they become irretrievably lost in anatomical bits and pieces. A limit beyond which Humpty Dumpty can never be put back together—at least, not perfectly. The body can never return to its pristine, original state after we've touched it with our hands. Eventually, my surgeon began to tell me not to get my hopes up. It was looking unlikely I'd ever operate again. Now our conversations ended with "We'll just wait and see." But what I saw was that there was little hope.

It's taken over a year for the bones in my spine to fuse. They did not heal fast or solidly enough. I took calcium, vitamin D, and many of the same supplements and herbs my patients once took. I scoured the medical literature and Internet—just as anyone else does—for every available alternative therapy to help my bones heal. I treated the incision with powerful magnets for half a year. Yep, I've even had a shark cartilage shake—once. It was ghastly. And there were times when the pain was so bad I thought I might lose my mind before I recovered. That has thankfully passed now.

My left leg cramps up. My foot flops clumsily against the floor. Sometimes it's too numb to tell if I placed it properly to fully support my weight. One leg's longer and stronger than the other. I spent a year and a half wearing an enormous metal-and-plastic brace that prevented me from inadvertently bending or jarring my bones while they mended.

I often walk now with a cane, in case my leg gives out. The "bag boy" helps me load groceries into the trunk of my car. Flight attendants politely urge me to board the plane early, ahead of the other passengers. I've learned to bear up under the stares of a hundred able-bodied folks who want to hurry past me on the escalator.

I was in a hurry once too. Now, whenever a sizable staircase looms ahead of me, I seek out the elevator. And I've learned how to ask for help, to get a hand, to be dropped off at the curb, and a thousand other minor insults that would once have hurt my pride. For such a long time, it was my technical and physical competencies that defined me and, now, I am just... well, just another patient.

I've also had to learn how to step down. To step down the stairs one step at a time. To step down as chairman of Surgery. And as the head of Neurosurgery. Seems reasonable that someone who doesn't perform surgery should not lead a Department of Surgery.

So I resigned my chairmanship. I was still a professor of surgery on the faculty, but at the time I was just able to shuffle a few steps using a walker. I needed to ask for help to wipe my ass. Not exactly the image of the invincible surgeon. Sometimes, when the ache in my back woke me up in the middle of the night, I'd break out in a cold sweat, wondering, Who the hell am I now? Now that I'm no longer a surgeon? It left me panicked. My wife would tell me I'm still her spouse. My kids would tell me I was still their father. But I had no answer for myself to the question of who I was.

Sometimes I contented myself that I might already have achieved more than most other surgeons. I'd risen faster than most. My career had just had a shorter duration. I'd compressed my career into one half of my working life. But then I'd hear myself say, So what? Why such a hurry to get ahead? Where did it get me? For more than a year, I just pitied myself. I felt broken, discarded.

On Halloween night 2004, I was attending a neurosurgical conference in San Francisco. I wanted to maintain my continuing medical education credits—just in case I might ever return to surgery, I guess. A significant number of folks were in the streets, in their elaborate costumes. As I was returning to my room at the Hotel Monaco, off Geary Street, I climbed on an elevator with a young couple under the full influence of the night's partying. The woman was dressed in an extremely tight, revealing nurse's uniform, spattered in fake blood. Her partner was dressed in surgical scrubs; he too was covered in way too much fake blood. As the doors of the elevator opened, the couple was in the throes of a deep, romantic kiss—I think she even had one leg curled up behind her as they smooched.

As I stepped onto the elevator with my cane, I jokingly asked, "How did the patient do?" looking at all the blood on their costumes.

The man disguised in the surgical scrubs jokingly answered, "I did everything I could. I just couldn't save him!" with exaggerated drama.

"Well, I know how that can feel. Have you gone out to break the news to the family yet?" I asked with feigned concern.

"No, I can't bring myself to do it," he said. "That's what my nurse and I were just talking about when you walked in."

"Ooh, you mean that passionate kiss?"

"Yeah, she was trying to give me a dose of courage."

"I know how that can be, buddy. I was a surgeon once."

"Really?" the man asked.

"Yeah...I was...I mean, am...I was a surgeon once...a brain surgeon."

Yeah, right. They both looked at me like I was some pathetic liar. But I was more struck by the tense: I *was* a surgeon, I had started to say. I should have said, I *am* a surgeon right away. But that's not how I really felt.

In the second year of my recovery, I started to take a renewed interest in redirecting my life. Just as a patient is a lot more than his ailment, I was learning to become more than just a surgeon. I began to ask myself, If I could focus my energies to change one single aspect about surgery, what would it be? I knew the answer to that question: I'd have to reinvent myself. That can take quite a while to accomplish. I had no more idea how to accomplish that than any of my own patients did. I'd have to take it one day at a time. But eventually an answer came.

Being a surgeon seemed to be in the past now, behind me, in another life. But some professions can hold their spell over you long after you've evolved into something else. For example, a writer can still be a writer even when working on something else. A priest, well, Catholics say, is always a priest—even if he renounces that life later. But a surgeon? That seems to fall more into the category of something you do. It's a state in which you live rather than something you become. Ask yourself: Is an opera singer still an opera singer after she loses her voice? Is a surgeon still a surgeon when there's no more surgery? And the surgical profession is not passive in this matter: No more surgery and it rejects you. You get the boot. Banned. Busted.

So what *could* I do? If there was one thing I'd change about surgery, I decided, it would be to eliminate the mistakes that hurt, maim, or kill patients. I decided to take a new step: I'd build a laboratory—a "think tank" where surgeons, researchers, and bioindustrial partners could look for new ways to reduce clinical and technical errors. I would create "a sandbox for doctors to put the *practice* back into medical practice." I would call it ASTEC—the initials would stand for the Arizona Simulation Technology and Education Center.

Over the next year, I recruited a team that was passionate about teaching the next generation of doctors to avoid making tragic, costly, and preventable errors. ASTEC began to thrive. In less than a year after opening, we had over a thousand individuals log more than 50,000 person-hours of training in the facility. We designed a whole new range of disposable, synthetic materials that permit surgeons and students to mimic procedures on any part of the body without ever needing any animal tissues. Students and residents could develop, practice, and refine their surgical technique in the ASTEC facility before they ever took a step into the operating room. I joined forces with faculty in engineering, computer graphics, and optics to create a whole new generation of surgical instruments.

We call them "smart" instruments because they can actually record and guide a surgeon's movements, and even warn a surgeon when the instruments drift out of range in the surgical field, endangering nearby organs. New computerized, image-guided technologies will soon permit a surgeon to visualize a three-dimensional holographic anatomic atlas that will appear to the eye to be superimposed onto the patient's body on the operating table. This kind of display will permit the surgeon to effectively "see" through the layers of the patient's tissues, letting important anatomical structures be visualized long before they could be inadvertently injured. A whole world of next-generation surgery now lies out there, in my imagination, and at my feet. Now I've been granted faculty positions in four different schools at the university, but Surgery is still home. Where my heart lies.

When I go to work at my office in the hospital, patients seem to smile at me differently from the way they did when I thought of myself just as a surgeon. Now I'm a guy with an ungainly limp and a cane. I'm just another one of the clumsy, awkward, struggling individuals who clutter the medical center's hallways. Just one of the broken folks. When I look at a fellow patient now, there's a different warmth in our mutual greeting. We're more alike than different: they're patients in search of doctor, and I'm a doctor searching for a patient. I'm completing a new phase in my surgical odyssey. I've passed over some invisible threshold—more patient than surgeon. I'm okay with that. Maybe even happier than I thought.

The word "patient" derives its meaning from the Latin adjective *patiens,* which literally means "one who endures." Patience is the only reasonable answer to all the questions we project out into the Universe from our quiet, mortal solitude: "Why? Why am I here?"

At first, the only response we receive is: Wait! Just wait! Wait patiently. Wait earnestly. Wait like a stone. Wait as long as it takes. Then wait some more. But the Universe has a soft spot for those who demonstrate they can endure. The heavens draw closer to those who show they can wait. Wait without pride. Without malice. They seek those who can sublimate themselves till they see their own life as a metaphor for the infinite ebb and flow of the galaxies. Patient souls are rewarded with a glimpse of interstellar patience, drawn in the dust from God's own hand.

The stars and planets do not care about the passage of time. They are deaf to the ticking of clocks. Time is a measure of human riddles. Death is only an illusion, a figment of time. The mortal tug we feel as patients arises from the paradox we feel between the timelessness of the galaxies and their yearning for intimacy, for reconnection with each one of us. The stars ache to reunite with us. They are affected by our capacity to connect with them. And as we call out, they struggle to answer us, to reply to our most sincere, sacred queries. We must wait till we are answered with their words of pure love. The mathematical cold of deep space is pierced by the passion of the stars to join with us. The heavens finally yield their language of unconditional love. With each one of us. For each one of us.

So being a patient has taught me to wait. With my whole heart. Endlessly. With no other purpose than to experience the waiting. Completely. In its entirety. I can cast myself into patience on a geological scale. I begin to hear the first murmurings of the Universe's voice. It is truly that of a mother calling out, beckoning to me. The voice is gentle. Sweet. Like music but beyond it. I must hush the beating of my own heart so I can hear the music coming from the stars. And then I do. They softly whisper, "You are our child." At last, they answer: "Yes." They sing, "You are our beloved. Truly. And forever."

Nada te turbe	*Let nothing disturb you,*
Nada te espante.	*Nothing frighten you.*
Toda se pasa.	*All things are passing.*
Dios no se muda.	*God never changes.*
La paciencia todo lo alcanza.	*Patience obtains all things.*
Quien a Dios tiene nada le falta.	*Whoever has God lacks nothing.*
Solo Dios basta.	*God is enough.*

—St. Teresa of Ávila, Spain
(1515–82)

Twenty Rules to Live By

So what conclusions can I draw from my experiences, these stories that I've shared with you? One feature binds all the tales together: every major surgery or illness is filled with moments of potential and even actual spiritual transformation. Health-related crises produce windows of vulnerability and susceptibility. They call into question everything we've achieved, pursued, or dreamt. A serious illness engenders a crisis of overwhelming doubt. But it can also become an opportunity for us: a chance for revelation, maybe unlike any other experience of our lives. The hospital can become a place of individual epiphany where both *attention* and *intention* can shift in an unsettling way. When life slams us off course, jars us off balance, we become most susceptible to the greatest changes from within. When the air is knocked out of us, we grasp the meaning of breathing.

Life-threatening episodes are terrifying. As the suffering patient, we're thrown into the empty, forbidding landscape of illness. Alone. No signs to point the way. Lost. Terror tugging at our soul. The hospital experience can influence both physician and patient. The patient, however, will really be the one in the crosshairs. At some point, the physician has to make a choice: remain uninvolved—the detached chronicler of the patient's course—or choose to be carried along by the patient's plight. Choosing the latter, there's always risk. Together, patient and physician must set out across a psychic and physiological wilderness.

All of us will one day endure this journey into the desert of sickness and death. How it affects us and changes us will determine whether we are to emerge with our own vision. The real magic lent to the medical arts comes from bearing witness to transformation.

It may be semantics to decide whether we see ourselves as part of a drama that is divinely derived or genetically derived. By either route of reasoning, God is probably the ultimate author. As mortals, we are left with a delicious dilemma: to accept or reject the notion of God's love. It is ironic that if God is the omnipotent Creator, then He must let us—His children—*feel* love ourselves. From us to Him. We cannot be ordered to love God. As powerful as God may be, no authentic love could exist between a human being and God without the freedom to *choose*. God's love may be boundless and everlasting, but each one of us alone must decide whether to declare it mutual. Whether to reject or embrace God. Either way, we will play our part while events unfold as they were meant to unfold.

Brent Curtis and John Eldredge, in their book *The Sacred Romance,* raise the issue of this poignant choice to love God:

> [God] can spin the earth, change the weather, topple governments, obliterate armies, and resurrect the dead. Is it too much to ask that He intervene in our story? But He often seems aloof, almost indifferent to our plight, so entirely out of our control. Would it be any worse if there were no God? If He didn't exist, at least we wouldn't get our hopes up. We would settle once and for all that we really are alone in the universe.
>
> —(THOMAS NELSON PUBLISHERS, 1997, p. 69)

I realize the futility of trying to steer anyone else's consciousness but my own in any new direction. Truth be told, I wrestle with my own spiritual ship. I hug the helm hard. I'm hardly qualified to give any counsel. Being a neurosurgeon certainly gives me no special privilege to dole out spiritual advice. And I freely admit that many experiences as a medical student and resident left me shaken with self-doubt. At times my own confidence abandoned me. On occasion, I felt as if I were playing in a game without rules or boundaries. There were no referees. No regulations. So like the shipwrecked schoolboys in William Golding's *Lord of the Flies,* I had to draw up my own rules. They helped me make better sense of patients' illnesses and guided my own behavior as a physician during my years as a medical student and resident. Most of the rules have been derived from personal experience rather than any special wisdom.

We've shared some of the most important and formative episodes in my life as a surgeon and a teacher of surgeons. I want to share some of my rules. None of them are unique, but they've stood the test of time for me. I hope that codifying some of them might make them more accessible to readers—patient or physician, student or pilgrim. My prayer is that these guidelines prove useful to you, those you love, and those you serve. In the end, the rules are meant to help you to "get a leg up," to find inspiration, and to make it back home after the trials and tribulations of disease.

Rule No. 1: Never underestimate luck—good or bad.

On the royal road to Thebes
I had my luck, I met a lovely monster,
And the story's this: I made the monster me.

—STANLEY KUNITZ, "The Approach to Thebes"

Luck is a personal monster. It's the dragon we all have to slay. We're called upon to do battle with luck—good or bad. There may be some truth to the notion that we make our own luck, lest that luck determine who we are now and who we may become. Each of us must learn to fit it into his or her personal vision of life.

Luck establishes the realm of what is possible; it sets limits to how we can respond to events and one another. Can we take credit for accidentally bumping into our mate, the partner of our dreams? Can we say we had anything to do with our choice of parents, or how they shaped us? Can we explain how one man dies suddenly from a heart attack at age forty-five, having jogged his whole life and eaten all his vegetables? And another, a chain-smoking alcoholic curmudgeon, lives till he's ninety years old and dies peacefully in his sleep? Can we justify the fact that some of us are born to privilege and comfort while others perish in the first few months of life for want of food and water?

The difference between being born into the First World or the Third is simply luck. Never feel any personal sense of triumph when you're lucky. Be grateful it went your way. Our sense of luck should bring with it a moral burden to see that equal opportunity, as far as possible, is eventually assured to one and all.

There's such a mercurial, intangible quality in luck. For example, one can see it in a fatal car crash. Often it's a drunk driver who suddenly veers across the median. He hits an oncoming minivan and kills an entire family. Some say this is God's work. Do we believe that God, the creator of Heaven and Earth, has an urge to be vindictive or capricious? Baloney. Albert Einstein remarked that he doubted that God would roll dice when it came to creating the universe, meaning that God could not be so whimsical as to play by the rules of chance. Creation is imbued with purpose.

I believe God looks on our human trials and tragedies with greater sadness than any of us can feel. In the Bible it says, "Are not two sparrows sold for a penny? Yet not one of them will fall to the ground apart from the will of your Father" (Matthew 10:29). God knows accidents are rampant in our affairs. For example, had that same family in the van been delayed a moment longer while the father had to hunt for his keys, then the van wouldn't have been there at that fatal instant. Had the drunken man's wife not left him for a rival that evening, he might not have been drowning his sorrows in alcohol, in that particular bar, at that particular hour. These connections between random events, a succession of "what ifs," can be traced as far back as we wish to go, right down to the time of Adam and Eve in the Garden of Eden. An infinitely long series of coincidences and events culminate in a moment of luck—good or bad. Either way it's instantly ours. We own it. It manifests as our personal monster.

When bad luck strikes, people curse. But when good luck hits, folks find reasons to explain it, why it might have been deserved, even due. And then the beneficiaries of good luck begin to think it was more than just accident. But it's the lack of an explanation, the deficiency of cause and effect, and the absence of malice or merit that make good luck such an embarrassment. Because we know no one is more deserving, more worthy than another to see that oncoming car swerve away and spare us. Which soldier deserves to hear the dull click of an enemy's dud shell. Which traveler has earned the magic deliverance granted by missing his connection to the flight that crashes.

It's when death veers away from you at the last second, when it gasps past you, missing you by inches, that you see what a freak accident life really is by its nature. Consider how you feel at that moment, when your life is inexplicably spared! Your heart pounds. As you shake from head to toe, sweet breath becomes a gift. No, you can't feel righteous at such a moment. You feel pure ecstasy, absolute relief. In this pivotal moment, life rushes at you like a tidal wave. It jerks you upward by the thin thread of mortality, holding you high above the abyss. Then it softly lets you down to earth. Instead of ending, life continues. You're alive, blessed with the greatest gift you'll ever receive—so rejoice! Give thanks!

But remember: Good luck is never ours to command. We are not its masters but rather its playthings. There's no more powerful ingredient that can be added to any patient's recovery process than the sheer astonishment of finding out you're still alive, of cheating death. While it's been said chance favors the prepared mind, good luck falls to those who respect it. My experience is that the happiest patients are also the ones who value luck.

Rule No. 2: Find a doctor who cares about you.

I'm usually dumbfounded when patients or their relatives confess that they really don't like their doctors. Worse, they have the impression that their physicians don't like them. What's with this? You feel that way about your physician but you're still going to let that person share life-transforming events with you? You're putting your very life in someone's hands, thinking that person doesn't care about you? It makes absolutely no sense.

So how will you know when you've found the right physician? Because that will be the one doctor who gives you the only opinion that matters. You'll understand that all the measured deliberations in the halls of medicine will never overrule or outweigh the significance of what your gut and your heart tell you. As Dr. Folkman pointed out at my medical school graduation, you need to find the one, true doctor in the house. As a patient, that one doctor is all you'll need. Once you've found him or her, stop. You're done. Jettison the rest. Let go of your fear and panic. Entrust yourself into that doctor's hands. Create your critical partnership, your kinship with that clinician. Your search is now over.

Rule No. 3: Never trade quality for quantity of life.

Cowards die many times before their deaths;
The valiant never taste of death but once.
Of all the wonders that I yet have heard,
It seems to me most strange that men should fear;
Seeing that death, a necessary end,
Will come when it will come.

So Shakespeare wrote in *Julius Caesar*. It takes courage to let go of life, especially the life of someone dear to us. We all know a handful of people for whom we would sacrifice our own lives if they could live—our children, a spouse, perhaps a best friend. We would lay our lives down without a moment's hesitation. So there are lives dearer to us than our own. If we accept that premise, then why is it such a leap for us to see there are circumstances where dying—especially quickly, heroically, and with dignity—is so much better than merely existing longer? I pray that when my time comes, I can pass from this life without struggle, without desperation. I hope I'll die bravely—and only once.

The answer to the question of whether a life should or should not be lived is heavily influenced by the quality of that life. But who measures that? Certainly only the individual who lives that life. No outside spectator is entitled to make that assessment. Quality is a personal yardstick. It can change over time and under different circumstances. If the will to survive continues to burn, then it is never the prerogative of the health care team to extinguish it for a patient. On the other hand, if a patient decides to "throw in the towel," then it's certainly not the physician's place to persuade the patient to accept further treatment in order to go on living. Living or leaving is, in a sense, the patient's ultimate call to make, and the physician's responsibility is to support whatever decision the patient chooses.

Rule No. 4: Live your life with death in it.

One of the major tenets of Buddhism is that attachment is the root of all suffering. It teaches us that only when we rid ourselves of our attachments will we experience pure joy and freedom. This is death's great, secret gift. We know that our own death is inevitable. We know that we will face a moment where we will leave this mortal existence. If we can focus on the significance of our own death, then we can learn to relish our physical life. Death becomes the key that unlocks the door where the beauty and meaning of every living moment can be found. If we espouse the goal of becoming "warriors"—individuals who live in full awareness—then we must learn to refine our actions under death's pressing reminder to live *now*. There can be no "would have done" or "could have done." There is only the desire to be—all in this single moment.

One of my favorite movies is *The Last Samurai*. The Japanese warlord Katsumoto tells the American, Captain Algren, "The perfect [cherry] blossom is a rare thing. You could spend your life looking for one, and it would not be a wasted life." In the final, climactic battle, as Katsumoto is dying, he exclaims, "Perfect.... They [the cherry blossoms] are all perfect." That is how someone, living with death on his shoulder, reminds himself of the exquisite and unbearable beauty of the present, of the very moment—even when it may be his last. We are fools when we let ourselves believe there's more time—a future lying ahead of us where we'll make changes, right a wrong, or correct our transgressions. The real truth—death's fundamental principle—is that our future is disappearing instantaneously, as soon as it appears. Hank Williams said, "We'll never get out of this world alive." The only way to be truly alive, then, is to embrace our own fatal adventure. That is how death teaches us to live.

As a surgeon, I've had lots of opportunities to observe individuals as they die. As I've talked to them, every one of my dying patients reports to me they feel a great sense of peace as death comes. They describe being in the midst of a beautiful, loving, divine presence. Close to the end, my dying patients appear to be overcome by a moment of final grace and rapture. There's a glorious light, they always say. There's a last, great overwhelming thrust of love propelling them across the chasm. I think that tells us what lies on the other side of this life, when we finally "pass over." I know it comforts me every single day of my life.

This has become one of the more important lessons I've learned as a physician. For me there is no surer evidence that something glorious and wonderful lies beyond our mortal existence. Death is not an end. It is a new beginning. It entails a magnificent reunion with God and all the wonderful souls that we've ever loved or will love. This is our destination when we pass over. Dying is not the end but rather a shift to a fresh form of life, a new and glorious manifestation of ourselves. In this regard, death would seem to be just another dramatic transition in a continuing cycle, similar in quality to birth. We jettison our mortal shell as we pass from one life form and consciousness to another, more wondrous than the last.

As Gandalf reports to Pippin in *The Lord of the Rings*:

"End? No. The journey doesn't end here. Death is just another path...one that we all must take. The grey, rainy curtain of this world rolls back and all turns to silver glass. And then you see it....White shores...and beyond. A far green country under a swift sunrise."

Rule No. 5: You cannot dodge the bullet with your name on it.

The emperor Napoleon is purported to have said to his doctor, "Our hour is marked, and no one can claim a moment of life beyond what fate has predestined."

I've seen patients go through an agonizing, destructive process of trying to "bargain" for their life. I wish I could ask them, in the midst of this dialogue, What if you already knew that your death was absolutely certain, that the moment was already inevitably, irrevocably written? Would you still struggle? Would you compromise your dignity? At some point, it will be your moment to die. No further bargaining. No despair. Your death is here.

So there's solace in Napoleon's observation. It is simply impossible to dodge or stop the bullet that is destined for each of us. It can take the form of cancer, a heart attack, a drowning, or a drive-by shooting. The way our lives will end is beyond our control. So we can give up trying to control it. We can loosen our grip. Instead of paranoid vigilance, we can substitute a calm awareness of our death's inevitability. Let death's inescapability be the source of our courage. We elevate our awareness by the knowledge of death—not by its rejection.

There's a distinction between letting death reinforce the meaning of life and "living every day as if it were your last." No one can really live that way without getting locked up. We cannot realistically approach each day as if it were our last. What would you do if you found out you were going to die at the end of this day? Would you go into work? Would you sit and pray? Would you run around in a panic trying to get out a last batch of letters or e-mails? Giving stuff away? I don't know exactly what any of us would do under such circumstances, but it's my guess that it would not feel too comfortable. It would make me feel utterly dejected. I wouldn't know where to turn first.

What we mean to convey is we should live fully but not finally. As the lyric to the song by the country-and-western band Rascal Flatts goes, "I want to be running when the sands run out." That's what we really mean. Keeping death in focus helps us live that way.

Rule No. 6: Ask your doctor to pray with you.

Sometimes patients feel guilty about wanting to pray before a major operation or during a major illness. They'll sheepishly admit, "I don't really believe. I never go to church anymore. So I'd be a hypocrite to ask for God's help now." Bull. God doesn't care if you had faith in the past. God cares about what you're feeling now. If you feel like you need faith and help, then it's time to pray.

There are a lot of docs who can't bring themselves to pray for help, so ask them to sit down with you and pray. Many are afraid they may look too vulnerable to their patients. They worry that praying makes them look weak and lacking in confidence. But what physician can't admit he or she could use help? We are all flawed human beings who cannot afford to reject God's help.

Don't be shy about asking family and friends to circle up with you in the hospital and join you in prayer. They'll bond with you or they'll stop visiting. Either way, you'll be better off.

Family and friends form the real circle of support we can always count on. This is our "tribe." These are our emotional relatives. While pulling everyone together in a circle, holding hands, may at first seem a bit contrived, it starts to feel just right after a short time. Our own circle of love is literally surrounding us, protecting us, sending its powerful, healing energies inward toward us.

I usually recommend that prayer circles be carried out as a "talking circle," where each person in turn is handed an object (it can be a feather, a stick, or an empty urinal; it really doesn't matter). The individual holding the "talking object" is the only one entitled to speak.

That person is allowed to share anything while a part of the circle. I usually have the patient in the hospital bed be the last one to hold the talking object so he or she can respond to everything that's been said by the other members of the circle.

This kind of circle can be a very powerful ceremony for every patient. It can also bring great solace to family members and friends who need to share some of their emotional burdens with the group. So significant is the emotional impact of the prayer circle if it is approached respectfully that it can change the course of a patient's illness.

Don't be afraid to ask the hospital chaplain, priest, or rabbi to stop by your bedside so you can talk and pray together. A severe, life-threatening illness should serve as an opportunity to open your heart further to God and your own spiritual awareness. As General Douglas MacArthur suggested when he said "There are no atheists in the foxholes of Bataan," there is no shame to be felt when the presence of pain, suffering, and death makes us want to get closer to God.

Ernest Hemingway wrote in one of his collections of short stories entitled *In Our Time:*

> While the bombardment was knocking the trench to pieces at Fossalta, he lay very flat and sweated and prayed, "Oh Jesus Christ get me out of here. Dear Jesus, please get me out. Christ, please, please, please, Christ. If you'll only keep me from getting killed I'll do anything you say. I believe in you and I'll tell everybody in the world that you are the only thing that matters. Please, please, dear Jesus."

The man is spared and the ferocious bombardment moves elsewhere. Hemingway adds ironically, "The next night back at Mestre he did not tell the girl he went upstairs with at the Villa Rosa about Jesus. And he never told anybody."

This passage has long stayed with me. It captures how despair can turn us instantly, even violently, toward God, and then we move on, maybe even forgetting how much we needed God's help in our time of crisis.

Rule No. 7: Never believe anyone who says "Nothing will go wrong."

Every time a physician invades the body with anything—a drug, a needle, even a suppository—there's some perturbation of the body's natural balance. The body is a divinely designed creation. It handles most disturbances very well. But no one can tell when the body is not going to respond in a predictable manner. Complications just happen. It's a fact of life.

Ask yourself this: How many of us have never had a car accident? Everyone has had at least one fender-bender in his or her driving career. How many of us have never received a traffic ticket? Practically no one. There's simply no situation in which anyone can guarantee that an accident or mishap won't happen. So any surgeon who tells you "nothing will go wrong" is either a fool or a liar, and probably both.

I remember a tragic case from my days as a neurosurgical resident. It involved a healthy guy in his mid-thirties. He was a father with three young children. He and his wife had decided that they were finished having children and that, as the husband, he should undergo a vasectomy for birth control. Their decision was entirely logical: the vasectomy procedure is a minor one and has a far lower complication rate and quicker recovery time than a tubal ligation in a woman.

He came in for the procedure. The surgery went perfectly, without a hitch. He returned to work the next day. On the third day, he began to experience increasing tenderness in his groin. The next day it was worse. He got an appointment to see his surgeon that same afternoon. When the doctor looked at the incision, it was getting infected. He put the young man on oral antibiotics and asked to see him in the office in two days. When the man returned, he had a full-blown infection in the groin, with red streaks of infection going up his abdominal wall and swollen lymph nodes on both sides.

The urological surgeon admitted the man to the hospital. He consulted an infectious-disease expert and put him on powerful antibiotics to control the infection. Despite everything being done aggressively and appropriately, the infection spread to the man's bloodstream. From there, the valves of his heart became infected. The patient's heart started to fail. He underwent emergency valve replacement. As the valve was removed, what we call "vegetations"—clumps of infected material on the edges of the valves—broke off and flew up into his brain. He developed a brain abscess (that's how I got to know him). He eventually died.

Now, when you trace this sad cascade of events, it all leads back to the original vasectomy. No one could have dreamt this poor man would expire as a direct result of a minor procedure. But it happened.

Finally, having a little superstition can help. If you say nothing is going to go wrong, then you've jinxed yourself. You've basically created an opportunity, almost a reason, for an accident to occur. Be humble. Be grateful. Good luck is a blessing.

Rule No. 8: Don't be turned into just another patient.

Hospitals have a way of making every patient look and feel the same. Patients slouch around in drab hospital gowns, towing IV poles, shuffling in sponge rubber slippers. Patients even start to smell the same, taking on the medicinal scent of the hospital. Like old vitamins and Lysol.

It's not good for any of us to become faceless, nameless patients. No one should be just the body that's in bed 448 with the hot appendix. Hospitals have a difficult time with rugged individualists. The last thing they want is *Homo indominatus*—a wild man. Hospitals don't want to struggle with our individuality. Be it a pair of pajamas or our favorite monogrammed bathrobe. Medical centers run on uniformity. They want every bed, every piece of clothing, every tray of food the same. That's what is easiest—for them.

Uniformity, however, is not good for living things. Life asserts itself by displaying variations. These are the traits that add color, texture, and excitement to existence. So I encourage you, as a patient, to fight back. Be an individual. Have your own favorite, comfortable clothing items in the hospital. Put up the photos of your kids. Bring that quilt your grandmother sewed. These are all talismans, sacred relics that remind you of your individuality. As the poet Dylan Thomas put it, we should all "rage, rage against the dying of the light." Last, our family and friends remind us how much we are cherished. They give us vivid cues, illustrating all we have to live for.

Rule No. 9: Listen to your favorite music.

I would not want to live in a universe where good could not ultimately triumph over evil. Or where there was no music. I simply cannot imagine a world without music. It's been said that "music is the language of the human soul." Music enlivens us. It injects emotional color. It can lend its energy to help you get better. And the beauty of headphones is that your favorite music choice won't bother anyone else.

Novel research from the musical therapy field has shown that patients' heart rates tend to synchronize themselves with the beat of music. One reason people find baroque music soothing is that its inherent rhythm of sixty-four to sixty-eight beats per minute is similar to that of a calm, relaxed heart. Music can be a powerful adjunct to the healing process. And music is one of the safest medicines you'll ever find. You can dose yourself as you please with no worries about toxic side effects.

I'm a big advocate of letting patients listen to music through headphones while they are asleep during surgery. It's been reported that such patients wake up more clearheaded and calm than other patients. It just makes sense to me that emerging from anesthesia into a world suffused with soothing music can only help a patient. I also advocate that families bring in compilations of a patient's favorite music and play it through headphones while the patient is in a coma or recovering consciousness.

Music works on us at a visceral, emotional level, and I want to harness all the positive energy I can to help my patients recover.

Rule No. 10: Never let hospital rules interfere with patient visiting hours.

Most hospitals want to scoot everybody out of the hospital at eight o'clock in the evening. Somehow families and friends get in the way after nightfall but are fine during daylight hours. There are also rules limiting children coming into the hospital. If you were recovering from a serious illness or surgery, wouldn't you want your kids to visit you? This insistence on restricting family access strikes me as potentially unhealthy, of removing support systems. Of course, all of these are subordinate to the patient's wishes.

If I had my way, I'd also permit dogs to be brought into the hospital. Horses. Parrots. Trained seals. Who really cares? How can the vitality lent to us by our beloved ones, human or animal, be cordoned off from us at the very moment we need it the most? Don't you think that I'll get better faster if one of my cherished dogs can sleep on my bed with me? Heck, yeah!

The Hotel Monaco is my favorite hotel in San Francisco. The reason I always stay there is they offer their guests a goldfish to keep in the hotel room. I find myself talking to the goldfish. That creature brings new life into my room; it becomes my companion, my hotel roommate. It raises my spirits. Not bad for being a little, two-inch-long fish.

Do you think a hospital is ever going to think like that? No way! They'll convene a committee of infectious disease experts along with a few stern-faced administrators to write a white paper predicting outbreaks of waterborne plagues and medical-legal nightmares of patients' feet getting lacerated by shards from broken goldfish bowls. A hospital will come up with a hundred "good" reasons why there should never be a goldfish in a patient's room.

That's why I recommend you get out of the hospital and go home as fast as you can. Outside the hospital, you start to take back control over your own healing environment. You can be with your dog. I will also tell you that whatever germs your dog may lend you by licking your face pale in comparison to the virulent, antibiotic-resistant bugs that flourish in our hospitals.

On a related note, I should add that in the Pediatric Ward, it is now accepted as much healthier for kids to have a parent stay in the room with the child than for the child to be alone. So if having family around 24/7 is not killing our kids in the hospital, how come we don't endorse it for all our patients? Finally, if you don't have a loved one "on duty" in the hospital during the night, who's on guard? Who's watching out for you? Monitoring what's happening?

As a surgeon, I'm reassured when I see family camping out at the hospital so they can stay with the patient. On the contrary, I start to worry when I see a patient who's alone, constantly unattended by family. That scenario, where no one is coming to visit, is a warning sign. That's a situation where I wonder, Who's going to help take care of these people's needs at home? On a professional level, I ask myself, If they're alone in this world, how strong is their will to live? The will to live is an essential ingredient of any recovery process and it is often tied to how well we feel loved.

Rule No. 11: The will to live is yours.

There's an old, awkward joke about a man who goes to visit his attorney. He wants to discuss how unhappy his wife appears to be recently. He's worried that she might be getting ready to leave him.

The attorney asks him, "Well, is your wife happy?"

The husband answers, "No, I don't think so. Come to think of it, she never smiles."

The attorney: "Well, go home and make her smile. Tell her some jokes."

So the husband goes back to his house and starts telling his wife jokes, one after another.

A week later the man comes back to see his attorney and says, "Well, my wife left me."

The attorney asks, "Well, did you tell her any jokes?"

The husband answers, "Yeah, and she told me she was unhappy but she was laughing all the way out the door."

The point here is that you can make people laugh and smile but you cannot make them happy. By the same token, if they're sad, disheartened, despondent—if there's nothing left to live for—no surgeon's skill can make them pull through or recover against their will. How often have we seen someone who seems to just wither away as soon as a lifelong spouse or companion dies? How often have we seen a person become completely "deflated," the way Rocky did in one of my earlier chapters, and just slowly and inevitably slip away? How many times have we seen someone die from a broken heart? No one else can live your life for you and no one else can give you the desire to live it. No one can give you the will to live.

Rule No. 12: Develop your own healing rituals.

As you can probably tell from some of my previous advice, I like my patients to take an active role in the healing process. They all should develop personal rituals or ceremonies to help themselves focus their energy on healing, on correcting imbalances from within. I don't care what the rituals are. Smudging. Crystals. Aromatherapy. Massage. Even candles (remember the Gypsy queen story). These rituals can be as mundane as praying and meditating each day or as creative as smearing bear grease and herbs on oneself (not on the incision, please).

Psychoneuroimmunology is an emerging scientific discipline that looks at how our emotional state can directly influence our physiology by augmenting or interfering with immune responses. All our leukocytes (white blood cells)—which fight off infection from bacteria, viruses, and foreign proteins—have receptors located on their outer surface specific for certain peptides. These peptides are molecules released from the brain that tell the rest of the body (and specifically our immune cells) how we are "feeling." Imagine for a moment you're going to be suddenly attacked by a prehistoric saber-toothed tiger. It might be a good thing to suddenly and aggressively activate your immune system in the event the tiger bites you. If you were to get an open wound, then you would need an augmented immune system to fight off infection. So nature developed a way for our emotional state to modulate our immune system.

Linking receptors on leukocytes to specific messenger molecules has evolved in our species to a considerable degree. Our immune system is particularly sensitive to a class of molecules known as "endorphins," a term that literally means "opiate from within." Endorphins are powerful opiatelike molecules that mediate pleasure and well-being in our central nervous system. When we are feeling happy, we secrete higher concentrations of endorphins than when we are depressed. When circulating endorphin levels are high, more molecules are fixed to the receptors on the leukocytes, activating white cells to fight off infection. If you're sad or depressed, there's less stimulation of white cells than normal and you literally become immunosuppressed. This latter fact may help explain why grief over the death of a loved one has such a profound impact on the morbidity and mortality of survivors.

This ability of white cells to be activated by circulating endorphins can be quite dramatic. In one example, a group of volunteers were shown lighthearted movies (mostly slapstick comedy) like Charlie Chaplin, Buster Keaton, and the Three Stooges. After they had been watching for several hours, a blood sample was taken. A second, separate group of volunteers were shown only horror movies, the kind of fare that makes your heart pound and gets you holding your hands over your mouth to suppress a scream. A blood sample from this second group was also taken.

The white cells from each group were then separated and placed in culture dishes where they had to attack bacteria presented to them on the culture medium. Guess what? The white cells that came from the folks who chuckled and watched the lighthearted movies could kill more bacteria than those cells that came from the people who watched the horror movies. Happiness makes for better immune function. The converse may also explain how someone succumbs to "voodoo" death. Or dies from a broken heart.

Rule No. 13: To heal quickly, avoid negative influences.

For almost my entire life I dreamed of having a ranch out West with horses. While I was a resident in Boston, I would regularly have lunch with a fellow surgeon named Ralph. He was a wonderful guy and we enjoyed swapping stories about our families. Over the years, Ralph and I grew to be close friends, and eventually I shared with him my dream of heading out West. But it seemed every time the subject came up, Ralph launched into a long list of all the obstacles that would make it impossible for me to achieve it. The first or second time this happened, I just shrugged it off. But I noticed that this pattern of serving up objections and obstacles became a habit—one that always left me deflated. Gradually, I found myself avoiding the lunches with Ralph. He was slowly poisoning my dream, and I needed it to sustain me through residency. After a while, I made a conscious decision to meet with Ralph only when I felt well defended and my ranch dreams were not on the table for discussion.

There are negative people and influences in our lives. Just because they are there does not mean we have to accept them. We must be aware of how and when negativity affects us. There's nothing wrong with deciding to avoid such negative "epicenters." Take responsibility for what you let into your heart. When we are sick, stressed, or sad, we become more susceptible to negative influences. At such times, we need to exclude those forces that do not raise our spirits. The simple rule of thumb is: Will this person make me feel better after he or she has visited me? Don't feel guilty for protecting yourself.

Rule No. 14: Don't let growing old make you crazy.

American culture is phobic about old age. In the next few decades, our society will experience the largest surge in the ranks of the elderly it has ever witnessed—a flood of baby boomers. Where will we put them all? How will we reshape the fabric of society to handle all these elders in our midst? I admit that I will be standing among them too.

How do we explain the fact that the elderly are regarded so differently in the Native American culture and Asian societies, such as in China, India, and Japan? In these cultures, the elderly are not rejected but revered. They are considered the crown jewel of any family or clan. The younger generations fight over who will be permitted to take care of the elders. Support of elders is considered the highest honor in a family, a sacred duty, for which one must be chosen. How different would our old age be, how altered our perception of infirmity, if our American culture saw our elderly in such a light? Instead of fearing banishment and imprisonment in so-called old-age homes, we might look to our families to honor us to the end of our days.

How did we come to loathe old age? To fear it? In part, I believe, it happened because we pushed the entire mutual, societal experience of death far away from our daily awareness. Think about this statistic: 95 percent of people polled express a clear desire to die at home. Currently, however, 90 percent of all individuals die in a hospital. Something's amiss here.

One explanation put forth is that hospitals are somehow better suited to deal with death. "They're equipped for it," we reassure ourselves. "Besides, how will we handle all that nursing care at home? What will the kids think? Take him to the hospital. He can die there." The result is that the experience of death has been eliminated from our lives. Many individuals have never seen a person passing away. I believe that our attitude toward old age, toward infirmity (and even disfigurement, for that matter) will not change till we discover a better way to incorporate death into everyone's experience. We will only "heal" this worry when we all fulfill our dream to die with dignity, at home, and surrounded by the ones who love us most. Choosing how we die is just as vital as how we live.

Rule No. 15: Never be dissuaded from alternative medicine.

Sir William Osler—one of my favorite literary and medical heroes—wrote about alternative medicine in 1910:

> I feel that our attitude as a profession should not be hostile, and we must scan gently our brother man and sister woman who may be carried away in the winds of new doctrine.
>
> —("The Faith That Heals," *British Medical Journal*, 1910; 1:1470–2)

Most physicians have an innate distrust of alternative and integrative medicine. Why are doctors so resistant to integrative medicine? I have no idea. As I discussed in an earlier chapter, there are valid reasons why integrative medicine has widespread popular appeal. First, we all seem to agree that whatever or however we feel internally can have a dramatic effect on our health. Everyone has felt that. A form of medicine, like integrative medicine, that appeals to our individual, personal experience (and validates it) should be attractive to all of us.

Second, there is a great suspicion in the lay public's mind that the medical profession has a vested interest in steering patients away from integrative solutions. Part of this distrust stems from physicians who are quick to condemn alternative medical therapies. They dismiss them without even hearing their possible merits. One major improvement in this "medical bias" is that the federal government has started funding (albeit at an embarrassingly meager level) research into alternative therapies. This could start to put integrative medicine on a more acceptable scientific footing in the eyes of traditionally oriented physicians.

The bottom line is that alternatives must be investigated when traditional, allopathic medical therapies prove insufficient. Physicians who dismiss alternative regimens are biased and closed-minded. I am generally suspicious that if they are so quick to dismiss alternative therapies, they may be just as biased with respect to *any* new medical therapy, no matter what the venue. A closed mind tends to remain so to *all* new ideas.

Rule No. 16: Never let a doctor determine your dignity.

There is so much about medical care that can be humiliating and degrading. I believe patients need to be strict with physicians as to what is or is not acceptable. I think too often we doctors just do things to patients because we know how to do them. How far a medical intervention should go is something better sorted out before we become ill. In the midst of a life-threatening crisis, it becomes difficult to stop events from just bulldozing ahead on their own momentum. Make your wishes known loud and clear.

I must point out to patients that "living wills" and "advanced directives" are virtually worthless, in my opinion. It's common for many patients to indicate that they do not wish "heroic measures" undertaken to sustain them. So, for example, if an individual indicates that he does not wish to be intubated and maintained on a mechanical ventilator, that still leaves much room for the discretion of a treating physician or next of kin. Did the patient mean that ventilation should never be employed? Or did he mean it could be used to treat a temporary condition like pneumonia but not instituted if the outcome might lead to a chronic, static condition where indefinite ventilation might ensue? And how certain should the treating physician be of the outcome? One hundred percent sure? Ninety percent? And if the outcome is undesirable, is the doctor empowered to withdraw ventilatory support? And under what conditions? In the final analysis, it's only family, next of kin (or those we empower by the means of medical power of attorney), who can be trusted to safeguard our dignity in the midst of a shifting medical landscape.

In this regard, I consider it vital for patients to undertake multiple, serial *premorbid* discussions with family and friends. Have these conversations before you become ill, before you're encumbered by hospitalization and illness. Try to envision a host of scenarios, as unpleasant as some of them may be. Be clear about your values, your concerns. Remember, you're providing future instructions, a map, about how and where you wish next of kin to proceed in the event that you can't make your own wishes known. This is obviously a serious undertaking. It can only be undertaken as an expression of mutual love and support.

Rule No. 17: Never let a doctor constrain your outcome.

Doctors can be very unimaginative—especially when it comes to predicting outcomes of particular illnesses or surgical procedures. Often they preface remarks about prognosis with qualifiers, such as "Most patients do not return to an active lifestyle." Or "You'll find that you have to limit many of your activities." Such "editorial" opinions plant a seed in the patient's mind about what he or she can shoot for and, frankly, they set the bar too low. Secondly, certain things may or may not happen to "x number of people under the large part of the curve." Remember: The truly "average" human being is a figment of statistical imagination. There is no such thing as an average person. And there should be no such thing as an average outcome.

I once had an acquaintance, who is a mathematician, explain to me the "subjectivity" of statistics: "Let's say," he argued, "there's a gunman on the roof of a building. Below it, you are standing as one individual in a crowd of one hundred people. You are told the gunman must shoot one of you to death. The odds of being killed are one in a hundred. The instant after the shot is fired, the odds are 100 percent for the individual who's hit. It did not really matter that, a moment earlier, his or her odds were 99 percent chance of surviving." By the same token, even if the odds of surviving an illness are only 10 percent, if you're among that 10 percent, your odds have just risen to 100 percent.

Every patient struggles with statistics. They seem to have become an integral part of describing almost every disease process. Asserted by retrospective series and cooperative studies, they become "the odds," the outcome, or the prognosis. They seem to spring from the scientific litera-ture like terrible wild beasts. The numbers can overwhelm the psychologi-cal defenses we have built to support ourselves through life-threatening episodes. Hearing or finding out about the statistics is often the worst part of learning about our illnesses. Patients need to hear the truth, but they also need to take comfort from this: Statistics mean *nothing* when it comes to a single person. When mathematicians try to consider one individual—the so-called *n equals 1*—all the statistical odds and pre-dictions become meaningless. Numbers can only inform us about popu-lations, massive groups of patients. The more individuals in the sample, the better the statistics. But they never can tell how *one single person* with a disease or surgical problem will fare. It is in that invalidation of statistics, in our mathematical singularity, that we can find refuge. When the numbers weigh upon us, we find sanctuary in our individual-ity. It exempts us from all the odds.

There's the heart of a champion in most of us. At the right time, under the right circumstances, we're all capable of delivering an "Olym-pic performance"—at least once in our lives. Remember a gold-medal athlete is crowned "the best in the world," not "better than average." So don't let a physician's casual comment squelch the "athlete" in you. Recovering from an illness or major surgery should engender the same discipline and dedication that athletes harness to return to their game. The best physicians encourage and exhort their patients just like a coach. Others often rain on your parade. Don't let them make you lose heart. Every patient wants his or her recovery to be exceptional—the best in the world. So don't be afraid to want it, to make it happen. My experience is that patients who believe they can cure themselves are usu-ally the ones who do.

Rule No. 18: Always ask a doctor what he or she would do.

Inquire how your doctor would react facing your same problem. What if it happened to someone he or she loved? This is the ultimate standard to apply to any medical care or therapy. So ask your surgeon, What would you do if you were in my shoes? Then stare him or her straight in the eye during the answer. If he or she looks away, something is going on. My advice is simple: If the doctor can't level with you about this, then how are you going to be able to proceed further? Go get yourself another surgeon.

Rule No. 19: Assign someone to be your guardian angel.

Having a guardian angel to watch over you is critical if you are the patient and want to get out of the hospital alive. Most folks have no conception of how prone the medical field is to mistakes. Research suggests that everyone who ever entered the hospital has been the victim of at least one or more errors while a patient. Fortunately, most mistakes are harmless. You weren't given your tray of food when you were first allowed to eat following surgery. You got one tablet of Tylenol instead of two. You were given the pair of slippers that belonged to another patient. Trivial issues but mistakes nonetheless.

The grimmer truth, however, is that the federal government estimates as many as 250,000 people a year may be killed in our health care system from adverse medical events. One review determined that over half of these mistakes are entirely preventable. All those in health care insist that they're doing everything possible to reduce errors, but they're not. Besides, human effort alone cannot reduce errors. Think about it. How safe would our air traffic control system be if it were just left up to an individual's memory or handwritten notes to ensure that aircraft did not collide? It would be a disaster. No, the aviation authorities long ago determined that sophisticated, computerized surveillance systems were required to guide and alert the human air traffic controllers to handle the complex variables in the skies.

To put the impact of such computerized systemwide surveillance systems into perspective, between the years 1980 and 1990, the aviation industry reduced aviation-related fatalities by more than 30 percent.

The likelihood of one individual dying in a fatal plane crash is less than one chance out of three million. Statistically speaking, a person would have to fly twenty-four hours a day, seven days a week, for four straight years to be at risk of a fatal crash. During that same decade, however, the fatality rate in the American health care industry rose by over 200 percent. The chance of experiencing an adverse medical event that will delay your discharge from the hospital is one in a hundred, and the chance of being killed outright by a mistake is close to one in a thousand! These are the terrible statistics darkening American medicine.

Many health care professionals protest that the profit margins for most hospitals and medical practices are so slim that no one can afford to invest in the kind of sophisticated systems we would need to make a dent in these tragic statistics of medical errors. But they do not point out that the cost of these health care–related mistakes is staggering: over 40 billion dollars a year. Reducing errors by even a small margin would more than pay to make American health care safe. Why won't anyone stand up and protest that this must stop and right now? The annual death toll from medical mistakes is equivalent to one 747 jumbo jet plunging out of the sky every single day of the year. How long do you think that would go on before government authorities would order all the jets grounded until the system was fixed? How many of us would be willing to take a seat aboard a 747 jet if the safety issues had not been addressed? Yet, like it or not, almost all of us have to go to the hospital, don't we? We can't become sacrificial lambs while we wait till the system is fixed.

So it's my advice to give someone in your family, a member who's smart and attentive, the assignment of writing down and recording everything that's done to and for you. I mean everything. They need to write down every question that arises. It's their job to make inquiries to the health care staff, to review medications, and to be a general pain in the ass. They need to keep meticulous journals or transcripts. They need to check every pill that's brought in to you. Ask, What's that little blue pill for? When's he supposed to get his next shot of pain medicine?

Aren't they going to hang up another liter of IV fluids before that one runs out? What time is that CAT scan scheduled for later today? When is the doctor supposed to be coming around to speak with us?

As I outlined earlier, something is screwed up with every single admission to the hospital. But the largest number of adverse events, by far, is caused by medication errors. So learn to question every single medication, every pill, every injection that is given to the patient.

I'll tell you about a near-fatal accident that occurred while I was an intern. There was a patient in bed 1 in a two-bed hospital room. It was his first postoperative day after an elective surgery, and orders had been written to start him on clear liquids and advance his diet as tolerated. The nurses decided to give him a cup of apple juice—always a favorite when you're on "clear liqs." The patient in the second bed was a "brittle"—one whose blood sugar can shift abruptly—a diabetic who had just undergone an amputation of his foot. This second patient was supposed to give a urine sample in a cup every four hours so the nurses could adjust his insulin dose by noting if he was spilling any excessive sugar into his urine. You can probably tell what's going to happen from here.

A nurse came in and set the apple juice next to the wrong patient, the one with diabetes. A second nurse came in and, seeing a cup half-filled with amber fluid sitting on the diabetic man's bedside table, assumed that it was the urine sample, grabbed it, and promptly dipsticked it. Of course, this cup contained the sweetened apple juice. The dipstick tape registered a dangerously high level of sugar. She became alarmed and left the room to draw up a substantial dose of insulin to treat the patient.

A third nurse now came in and found the diabetic man's cup of urine sitting outside the room, next to the first man's hospital chart. She saw the order written for apple juice and assumed that this must be the apple juice the patient in bed number 1 had requested. She brought the cup and placed it next to the patient on his bedside table. The second nurse came back and put a large dose of insulin into patient number 2's intravenous line. Of course, the diabetic gentleman went into insulin shock just as patient number one suddenly spat out the first foul-tasting mouthful of his roommate's urine. Just always assume somebody, somewhere along the line, is going to screw up.

Don't be afraid to make a pest of yourself. Remember, it's the squeaky wheel that gets the grease. If the physician and nursing staff know that someone's watching vigilantly, they will pay more attention. It's just human nature. Ask yourself: How many of us continue to speed once we see that a police patrol car's parked on the side of the road? No one! We all step on the brakes and slow ourselves back down to the speed limit. It works the same way in the hospital.

Rule No. 20: There's *no* surgery like *no* surgery.

Surgery remains the "court of last resort" when less invasive and less dangerous medical therapies will not work or just fail. I don't believe in most "prophylactic" surgeries, because there are just too many accidents that can happen. Often what you are trying to prevent with the surgery is exactly the complication you may get. For example, a patient is found to have a bulging cervical disk. The surgeon recommends having a discectomy, because "you never know, you might just get paralyzed if you have a car accident." So the patient consents to having the disk in his neck removed. Just in case.

The unthinkable happens: There's unexpected manipulation and trauma to the spinal cord during the surgery. The disk is out but the patient wakes up paralyzed. Or you try to fix someone's face so that he'll look younger, but there are complications. A serious infection sets in, leaving the patient disfigured. Again, is cosmetic surgery reasonable when it's framed in the light of potential mishaps? Like it or not, surgery's a crapshoot—for both the patient and the surgeon.

So when should a person consent to having surgery? One of two circumstances has to be met before proceeding with an operation. First, is your *life* in direct and imminent danger? Let's say you're diagnosed with cancer. You have to have it removed. In a perverse sort of way, this makes the decision straightforward. If there's a higher likelihood that you'll die without the surgery, then it's worth the gamble. Raise the favorable odds even more by letting only an experienced surgeon perform the procedure. Then, as they say in the casinos, *Les jeux sont faits*. All the bets are in and it's time to put your faith in God and your fellow man. Take the plunge, because whatever is meant to happen will. And pray too.

The second condition is much trickier. It's harder to know if this condition is really being satisfied. Ask yourself: Is my *lifestyle* seriously threatened without surgery? For example, you have a bum knee. It's interfering with your active lifestyle. You can't go on hikes. There's too much discomfort to play tennis or go for a bike ride anymore. The dysfunctional knee won't kill you, but how much will you enjoy life without getting it repaired? So who makes that call? You do. This is the gray area where a surgeon can advise you about options—can try to lay out the odds—but only you can know how you want to live. And only you know how much you're willing to risk to live the life you want.

Acknowledgments

No one accomplishes anything in this life on his or her own. Even when we stare in awe at what might appear to be a solitary feat—like climbing to the top of a mountain alone—there is invisible support. There are loved ones at home who cherish the adventurer. A mentor to teach. A colleague with whom the experience can be shared. And unseen magic too.

As I put these stories together for this book, I was struck by the enormous debt I owed to so many. There were recollections of patients, family, and colleagues that left me giddy with joy. But others left me—often at the same time—in tears. I have been the recipient of so many gracious turns and favors, too many of which are debts I cannot repay because the parties to whom I owe so much have already departed this life. Still, I feel better for the effort of just trying to list them here. Only they know the full extent of the debt I owe them and how great my gratitude will always be toward them.

First, I want to thank my grandfather. He provided me with my first opportunity to see a complete man: sophisticated, cultured, erudite, and—above all—brave. He was—is—someone who is hardly out of my daily thoughts for more than an hour. He infected me with his love of books, horses, and bygone days of nobility and its heroes. He was—as every grandfather should be—bigger than life. He was the first person to encourage me to write and keep a journal about my daily thoughts and experiences—something I have done faithfully from the age of sixteen to the present. That journal is now some twenty handwritten volumes in length and the source of much of my recollection and reconstruction for many of the stories in *The Scalpel and the Soul.*

The second person to whom I am most indebted is my wife, Janey. I had the great fortune of finding my wife when she was only nineteen years old and I was twenty-two. I had to wait until she graduated from college before her parents would let me marry her. We've been together ever since, for more than thirty-five years. Stephen King, in his marvelous book *On Writing,* states that every author writes with only one reader in mind—"the first reader." This is the person the writer envisions reading the pages as they are born, first written. My first reader is Janey. She has filled my whole life and those of our three grown children with her shining presence. She is the sun in our family's universe.

To my children, Josh, Luke, and Tessa, I owe a great debt: becoming and being a neurosurgeon made me miss a great deal of their lives. I hope that as I become older and wiser, I may try to make up for those absences in some small way. My children are, in the end, the most meaningful experiences in my life.

There is my mother, Lilli, and my brother, Patrick, who always created a home in their hearts when life seemed to offer none.

I also need to acknowledge a few mentors. Wilder Penfield was the neurosurgeon who inspired me to go into the field of neurosurgery. Daniel Federman, the dean of students at Harvard Medical School, refused to let me settle for anything but the most rigorous training as a neurosurgeon.

Massachusetts General Hospital was my home, my country, and my family for eight years. I received within the halls, the wards, and the operating theaters of MGH the finest training I could ever dream of as a physician. It was at MGH that I also found some of my greatest inspirations. There are a few I would like to thank.

Peter Black, in whose lab I learned the fundamental principles of scientific investigation. Peter combined an encyclopedic intellect with a profound sense of philosophy. Roberto Heros was my neurovascular mentor. No surgeon more epitomized for me the dashing courage and unshakable confidence that a brain surgeon must exhibit. Roberto also had a big heart—one big enough to help me find the true joys of surgery. There is Bob Ojemann. To my mind, he's the greatest neurosurgeon I ever met. He was the ultimate craftsman and tackled the most difficult and daunting surgical cases with superb, extraordinary outcomes. Dr. Ojemann showed me that the best teachers could spur you to greater heights by inspiration rather than by intimidation. Then there is Nicholas T. Zervas, the chairman of the Neurosurgical Department at MGH. He had an encyclopedic knowledge of the neurosurgical literature that he combined with a very humanistic, compassionate approach to his patients. It was Dr. Zervas who cautioned me early in my career, "It is better to die by the hand of God than the hand of man"—something I always remind myself about when considering life-threatening surgery for any patient of mine.

I made many lifelong friends at MGH, including David Frimm, Rich Ellenbogen, Karl Swann, Fred Sonstein, Kevin Kiwak, Kevin McGrail, Brian Beyerl, Eric Zager, Fred Barker, Chris Ogilvy, Joe Madsen, Joe Phillips, Jim Schumacher, Bill Butler, Andrea Halliday, and a whole host of other surgeons, far more gifted than I, who have included me in their midst.

At the University of Arizona, there have also been many colleagues: Milos Chvapil, who was the director of Surgical Research; Bruce Jarrel, the surgical chairman before my tenure in that job; Phil Carter, my neurosurgery chief when I arrived in 1990. And then colleagues: Martin Weinand, Karsten Fryburg, Bill Smith, Joel McDonald, Mitch Gropper, Gabriel Gonzalez-Portillo, Miguel Melgar, John Porter, Mike Demeure, Hugo Villar, and a host of surgeons, many of whom I have had the honor to recruit. Jim Dalen was the dean of the College of Medicine while I was the chairman of surgery and epitomized the kind of leader at whose feet one is honored to lay his sword.

I would also like to express my gratitude for my most recent colleagues: the team members in the Arizona Simulation Technology and Education Center: Mohamed Salkini, Alyson Knapp, and Jo Marie Gellerman.

I have treasured my close friendship over many years with Richard Carmona, until recently the surgeon general of the United States. I had wanted Rich to become my vice chairman of the Surgery Department. I was shocked to receive a call from Andrew Card, the chief of staff at the White House, telling me the president of the United States was also trying to recruit Rich. The president won. Rich is a man of inestimable integrity, strength, and courage. He and his wife, Diane, are sources of constant inspiration to me.

Within my sphere as a writer, there are many people to whom I am indebted. First, there is Rod Serling, the creator of the television series *The Twilight Zone*. Rod was my creative writing teacher for two years at Ithaca College. It was one of the luckiest breaks in my life to be so close to such a great writing talent. Rod had a profound love of the writer as storyteller and introduced our class to some of the "greats" in science fiction: the two most memorable for me being Harlan Ellison and Ray Bradbury.

I am blessed with many wonderful friends in Tucson. First, there is Michael Karopatkin of Spectra Consulting. Michael was the first to encourage me to think about writing a book. My beautiful friend Brian Walker never once faltered in his belief that I could offer something back to the surgical profession—from the heart. I cannot express how much I have learned about the art and craft of writing from Rebecca Salome. She combines a love of writing with an ability to dissect what it takes to make a writer speak from the heart, with an authentic voice. I could not survive without the expert skills of my administrative assistant, Carol Shaughnessy-Quinn. She is all things: sergeant major, transcriber, editor, confidante, and coach. Most of all, she surmounts the quirks of my obsessive personality and the emotional tempests that sometimes sweep over me, and gets the job done.

My literary agent, Mike Larsen, is not only willing to take chances on first-time authors but also loves books enough to find more. Dottie DeHart, my publicist, has demonstrated an enduring faith in the mission of so many of the writers she champions: to infuse spirituality back into people's personal lives. My editor, Mitch Horowitz at Tarcher/Penguin, is the embodiment of what every writer imagines a good editor should be. Mitch can make an inquiry into the details of choosing a particular word or piece of punctuation, but can also ask an overarching question or suggestion that makes me aware that I have not fully expressed what I intended. He believes passionately in taking on projects that connect the spiritual with the scientific because he shares a longing to look beyond the physical world for the most enduring answers to the questions life raises. Mitch is also unafraid to be a fan of his writers' work. He inspires an energetic, devoted team. Shanta Small and Laura Ingman, from the publicity team at Penguin, impressed me not only with their professionalism but also with their genuine enthusiasm and familiarity with my book—one among the hundreds coming across their desks. I was touched that they cared so personally about what I had written.

I need to express my gratitude for my friend and colleague Andrew Weil. Andy has never wavered in his support for me as I developed a collection of "medical stories." From the very first, he offered to write a foreword to my book—even when I was not sure I had the workings of a book. Andy has always been an inspiration to me. Before Andy became a well-known author and speaker to the outside world, he was already famous within the University of Arizona for making himself available to help colleagues and their patients find alternative methods when others in the medical profession had given up and were no longer willing to offer help or hope. He has always stood for intellectual courage and honesty in medicine, patiently championing the value of integrative medicine, even when it was very unpopular with so many of his peers, in both allopathic and alternative schools. Andy has managed to lead a major movement to revolutionize how we think about health and healing without developing that worst of all leadership traits: telling others what to think or believe. He has always valued the ability of both patient and physician to judge the merits of therapy on their own. I am forever in his debt.

Last, there are my patients and their families to thank. First, for sharing their lives and perils with me. Second, my patients have always managed to coax me into becoming a better man and physician than I thought I could be. I have always thought that God wanted me to become a surgeon because He knew that without my patients, constantly reminding me of what is good and important in life, I would have gone astray long ago. My patients have always shown me the truth that lives and shines at their bedside. I will hold them forever in my heart for showing me the way.

About the Author

Allan Hamilton is a Harvard-trained brain surgeon. He currently holds four professorships at the University of Arizona: his primary appointment as professor of neurosurgery, as well as also being a professor in the Departments of Radiation Oncology and Psychology and the School of Electrical and Computer Engineering. He and his wife, Jane, own a small ranch on the outskirts of Tucson, where they once raised three children and now raise Lipizzaner horses and Brangus cattle. They conduct horse-training and equine-assisted learning clinics around the United States and Europe.